W9-BAO-096

The Hemochromatosis Cookbook

Also by Cheryl Garrison

The Iron Disorders Institute Guide to Hemochromatosis

The Iron Disorders Institute Guide to Anemia

Exposing the Hidden Dangers of Iron

*Encyclopedia of Civil War Usage: An Illustrated Compendium
of the Everyday Language of Soldiers and Civilians*

The Hemochromatosis Cookbook

Recipes and Meals for Reducing the Absorption of Iron in Your Diet

CHERYL GARRISON

CUMBERLAND HOUSE
AN IMPRINT OF SOURCEBOOKS, INC.®

A portion of the proceeds received from the sale of this book will be donated to the Iron Disorders Institute.

THE HEMOCHROMATOSIS COOKBOOK
Published by Cumberland House Publishing, an imprint of Sourcebooks, Inc.
P.O.Box 4410
Naperville, IL 60567-4410
www.sourcebooks.com

Copyright © 2008 by Cheryl Garrison

All rights reserved. Written permission must be secured from the publisher to use or reproduce any part of this work, except for brief quotations in critical reviews or articles.

Cover design: JuliesRulesDesign
Cover photograph: Justin Lightley / GettyImages

Library of Congress Cataloging-in-Publication Data

Garrison, Cheryl D.
  The hemochromatosis cookbook : recipes and meals for reducing the absorption of iron in your diet / Cheryl Garrison.
    p. cm.
  Includes bibliographical references and index.
  1. Hemochromatosis—Diet therapy—Recipes. I. Title.

  RC632.H4G375 2008
  641.5'631—dc22

2008014800

Printed in the United States of America
VP 19 18 17 16 15 14 13 12

To my son David and three women who taught me about the benefits of good nutrition: Naoma Goben, Elsa Blanton, and Irene Tate

———————————————————————

I wish to thank people who made this book possible: publisher Ron Pitkin, editor Lisa Taylor, designer Julie Pitkin, and contributors Gene Weinberg, Gerry Koenig, Peggy Clark, David Garrison, Jen Opperman, Mark Princell, Richard Passwater, Carol Bates, Chris and Harry Kieffer, Art Callahan, Chip Sullivan, Jane DePew, and Adam Tanner.

Contents

Hemochromatosis Cookbook

Foreword

It's ironic! For decades in the United States there has been an intensive educational program urging people to eat foods rich in iron, mainly red meats. For the more than one million Americans who unknowingly have iron overload disorders, however, that is bad advice. Furthermore, there is no educational program to warn people of this deadly problem. Erroneously, most authorities still believe that iron overload disorders are rare. I wouldn't call a deadly disease that affects more than a million Americans "rare."

Iron is vital for the transport and utilization of oxygen, so much so that it may be said that a partnership exists between the two which requires maintaining a balance. We often hear that iron deficiency can be a problem for about 10 percent of toddlers, teenage girls and women of childbearing age in the U.S., and for more than one billion people worldwide, according to official estimates. It's very common for nutritionists and physicians to recommend that people with poor or questionable diets take iron supplements without even testing for iron deficiency. However, few people realize that dietary iron is contraindicated for about 1 in every 250 Americans.

It's not that these people eat too much iron, but that they have a genetic abnormality that causes "iron overload disorder." As many as 1 in 9 Americans carry one of the genes that can lead to the disorder. This makes it the most common known genetic disorder in the U.S. It is now believed that even having one of the two genes may, in some cases, lead to an iron absorption abnormality.

The problem is compounded by the fact that possibly between 1 million and 1.5 million Americans have undetected iron overload and do not become aware of their deadly disease until it is too late. The symptoms, such as fatigue and depression, are common to a number of ailments, which are, unfortunately, too often confusing to physicians, who are taught that iron overload disorders are rare genetic diseases. Actually, as already mentioned, hereditary hemochromatosis is the most commonly inherited disease. Because most physicians still believe that iron overload disorders are rare, one-third of hereditary hemochromatosis (the worst form of iron overload) patients in one study reported that they had to see an average of eleven physicians before they were correctly diagnosed, and one-fifth reported that this process took ten years.

Fortunately, *The Hemochromatosis Cookbook* helps clarify the problem. It provide an easy-to-understand explanation of the science behind the iron overload disorders and presents practical and expert advice on how to deal with these disorders. Making the more than two hundred recipes in this book part of their dietary plan will no doubt help those who suffer from iron overload disorders.

—Richard Passwater, Ph.D., Director,
Solgar Nutritional Research
Center, Berlin, Maryland,
and Vice President of
Research, Solgar Vitamin
& Herb Co., Inc.

Preface

The Hemochromatosis Cookbook is the second edition of our very popular book *Cooking with Less Iron*. This edition contains over two hundred recipes and an eating plan for those who are trying to manage iron intake and excess body iron levels. Because diabetes mellitus is often a consequence of hemochromatosis, some tips for those with this condition are included in this edition.

I first learned what excess iron can do to the body when my son David, who was sixteen at the time, became very ill. He had lost forty pounds in a short span of time, was profoundly tired, had joint pains, and his skin had turned an ashen gray-green color. Blood chemistries revealed a "wildly" high iron level, elevated blood sugar, and rising ferritin. Juvenile diabetes was suspect. When I asked about the high iron, the doctor remarked that "high iron goes along with diabetes."

Today, we know that high iron is a risk factor for diabetes, but back then, it did not make sense to me. David's symptoms were not typical of diabetes—they seemed to fit better with juvenile arthritis. I needed answers—but everything I read about high iron in medical books was accompanied by the word *fatal*.

Emotional and scared for my son's life, I turned to the Internet, which only made matters worse. After reading posts from people who seemed experienced with iron overload, I became convinced that my son had cancer and that I needed to run out and get genetic tests—something I regret doing, mostly because my actions were driven by fear rather than knowledge. Once I calmed down and began reading with a healthy skepticism, I realized how easily fear can cloud one's judgment, especially when the health of one's child is at stake. Genetic tests are extremely helpful when a person is fully informed and counseled about how to interpret the results; however, a genetic test tells you nothing about your iron levels, only that you may be a risk for iron loading caused by mutations of the HFE gene.

It became my passion to find out what was making my son sick and to get him well. I also wanted to share my knowledge with others who faced similar fears. Today, the Internet is a wealth of information, but a person needs to know how to qualify some of the things they read on the Net. Through the IDI websites, patients have access to tools I wish I'd had when I first began my research on iron overload:

helpful record-keeping forms, books, pamphlets, newsletters, information about patient-to-patient online excess iron discussion group, access to patient-to-expert online forums and websites filled with solid, medically sound information. As for the diet, one does not have to become a fanatic about the iron content in foods or what one eats or cooks in. Before eliminating nutritious food choices from the diet, read some of the myths about iron; know the consequences of overdoing things and taking risks with unhealthy approaches to controlling iron balances.

My sincere hope is that this book will help to broaden your knowledge about iron and make sensible, not emotionally charged, choices about diet and behavior.

—Cheryl Garrison, executive director and a founding director
of Iron Disorders Institute (IDI)

The
Hemochromatosis
Cookbook

Introduction

As a physician it is rewarding when a diagnosis can be accompanied by hope. Such is the case with early detection of hereditary hemochromatosis, a leading cause of iron overload disease.

Hereditary hemochromatosis (HHC) is a genetic disorder of iron metabolism. It is not a blood disease. A person cannot catch hemochromatosis; it is inherited from their parents. Persons with HHC have a defect somewhere in the absorption process. This causes them to take in excessive amounts of iron from their diet. Iron cannot be excreted, and after several years time this excess iron accumulates in vital organs such as the liver, heart, pancreas, joints, and brain. Iron-loaded organs cannot function properly and the result can be disease, such as diabetes, liver disease, arthritis, depression, impotence, infertility, or premature death from a heart attack.

When detected early, HHC can be treated and dramatically reduce a person's risk of developing these serious and chronic diseases. Hemochromatosis is a condition we physicians can do something about. We can suspect it in anyone because it is common: 1 in 250 Americans are believed to have genetic hemochromatosis; nearly 30 million are believed to be carriers. Physicians can suspect HHC in anyone with a history of chronic disease, especially when a parent has died prematurely. Doctors can identify it early because it's real; with the discovery of HFE, the gene for hemochromatosis, the condition, once thought to be rare, was validated as real and prevalent among Caucasians. Also, HHC is easily detected. Two simple blood tests, serum ferritin and transferrin iron saturation percentage, can reveal elevated tissue iron levels. Physicians can also use genetic analysis to detect HHC, especially in families where one case has been diagnosed. Doctors should inform families about HHC because it can kill. Undetected and untreated hemochromatosis is one of the greatest risk factors for chronic disease, which can lead to death at an early age. The mean age of death from heart attack in undiagnosed males with hemochromatosis is estimated to be age fifty-eight; for females it is believed to be age seventy-four.

When I diagnosed my first case of hereditary hemochromatosis there was very little information about the disorder. Except for treatment using aggressive phlebotomy, there was nothing to help a physician guide a patient in the management of their iron imbalance. Diet guidelines were nonexistent or too extreme. Through organizations such as the Iron Disorders Institute and its educational publications, we now have more to offer patients with HHC. We have learned about the problems associated with over-bleeding, how to determine reaccumulation patterns, that tobacco smoke is loaded with iron, and that certain foods inhibit or enhance the absorption of dietary iron. With this knowledge, it is clear there are preventive measures that can help control the absorption of the metal. This information can be vital to a person with an iron loading disorder such as hemochromatosis.

Careful monitoring while deironing, especially during the final phase, compliance with therapy, and controlling one's diet, are key to managing hemochromatosis. In *The Hemochromatosis Cookbook* Cheryl Garrison has combined her years of experience as an educator, her knowledge about iron imbalances, and her practical experiences as a restaurant owner to create a simple and helpful eating plan for persons with HHC. Anyone with excessive tissue iron can benefit from the recipes and helpful tips in this book.

Talk with your physician about hereditary hemochromatosis. Contact the Iron Disorders Institute for literature about the disorder and visit their website at www.irondisorders.org. Meanwhile, keep your iron levels in balance, eat right, kick the tobacco habit, and enjoy life!

> —*Mark Princell, M.D.,*
> *Spartanburg Regional Health Systems,*
> *Spartanburg, South Carolina*
> *Iron Disorders Institute Medical and*
> *Scientific Advisory Board Member*

Why Cook with Less Iron?

Individuals with hereditary hemochromatosis absorb up to four times more iron from the diet than do people without hemochromatosis. Cooking for reduced iron *absorption* can help a person manage iron intake when iron levels in the body are too high.

The body has no natural way to excrete iron excesses, and over time the metal accumulates to toxic levels in vital organs such as the liver, heart, pancreas, brain, pituitary gland, bone marrow, and joints. People with high iron levels are at an increased risk for premature heart attack, diabetes mellitus, arthritis (osteoarthritis), bone disease (osteoporosis), liver disease, and hormone imbalances such as hypothyroidism, hypogonadism, and adrenal problems. These hormone imbalances can result in many symptoms, including depression, loss of sex drive, infertility, or impotence. Maintaining a healthy iron balance in the body can lower the risk of developing chronic disease and premature death.

Iron is an essential nutrient; human beings cannot survive without it. Functioning normally, iron carries life-saving oxygen to cells, where it picks up carbon dioxide and delivers it safely to the lungs to be exhaled from the body. Without iron, we suffocate and die; with too much iron, we rust and die.

For hundreds of years the medical community has focused on iron deficiency anemia, which remains a critical health issue today throughout the world. Before the 1996 discovery of HFE, the hemochromatosis gene, many health policy makers and physicians thought hemochromatosis was rare—an older male's disease. At that time only a handful of scientific journals reported the suspected prevalence of hemochromatosis. Since that time, however, a proliferation of reports have been published about the dangers of too much iron in the body. The more we learn about excess iron, the greater the need becomes for more research to better understand the factors that drive the HFE gene, such as hepcidin, receptors, ferroportin and other proteins. We also need increased awareness about the consequences of late detection and absence of treatment for iron-loading conditions such as hereditary hemochromatosis.

Frequently Asked Questions (FAQs)

What is hemochromatosis (HHC)? There are five known types of hemochromatosis. The most common is type I or classic hemochromatosis. This type is an inherited metabolic disorder that results from excessive amounts of iron in the body.

Who is at risk for type I hemochromatosis? The Centers for Disease Control and Prevention (CDC) estimates that one million Caucasians have the genetic makeup for classic hemochromatosis.

How is the excess iron removed? For most hemochromatosis patients, treatment is therapeutic phlebotomy, which is the same as a blood donation, except a doctor's order is required because blood can be removed in larger amounts and more frequently than routine blood donation.

How do I know if I have iron overload? Many people think that high hemoglobin means iron overload. Though hemoglobin values are extremely important in body iron management, hemoglobin alone does not demonstrate a person's body iron levels. Two other tests are needed: serum ferritin and transferrin iron saturation percentage (TS%). These tests are best done fasting, that is, nothing by mouth except water after midnight or prior to bloodwork. Normal range for TS% is 25 to 35 percent. Normal ranges for ferritin differ according to age and gender. Note: some hemochromatosis patients can have elevated hemoglobin, but generally the cause is not due to high body iron but rather to smoking, being underhydrated, or some other condition, such as polycythemia vera.

Can a person have both anemia and iron overload? Yes. Some examples of conditions in which a person can have anemia with iron overload are: G6PD (glucose-6 phosphate dehydrogenase enzyme deficiency), sideroblastic anemia,

Important Ferritin Reference Ranges	ferritin	Adult Males	Adult Females
	Normal Range	up to 300ng/mL	up to 200ng/mL
	In treatment*	below 100ng/mL	below 100ng/mL
	Ideal maintenance	25-75ng/mL	25-75ng/mL
Adolescents, Juveniles, Infants & Newborns of normal height and weight for their age and gender			
Male ages 10-19 23-70ng/mL		Infants 7-12 months 60-80ng/mL	
Female ages 10-19 6-40ng/mL		Newborn 1-6 months 6-410ng/mL	
Children ages 6-9 10-55ng/mL		Newborn 1-30 days 6-400ng/mL	
Children ages 1-5 6-24ng/mL			

Chart reprinted with permission from Iron Disorders Institute, 2006
*having therapeutic phlebotomies

chronic hemolytic anemia, thalassemia, sickle cell disease, myelodysplasia (MDS), and cancer. In these cases, the iron overload is caused by repeated, early break-down of red blood cells or repeated blood transfusions. Excess iron for people with anemia must be removed by drugs specifically formulated to bind with iron and remove iron. In our book *Guide to Anemia*, we address these conditions and the treatment.

Can a person with hemochromatosis also be iron deficient? Yes. People with hemochromatosis can be overbled (too many phlebotomies, too close together) and become so severely iron deficient that they have to consume iron to get better. There are also cases of hemochromatosis patients who, when diagnosed early, panic about the potential of high stores (ferritin) and go to extremes with their diet and supplements, making themselves severely iron deficient.

How do I know if I am iron deficient? Your doctor can measure hemoglobin, serum ferritin, and transferrin iron saturation percentage (TS%). For people with hemochromatosis, all three tests are important. Hemoglobin measures functional iron, that is, what you have working to maintain the body's oxygen and carbon dioxide levels. Serum ferritin demonstrates the amount of iron you have in storage. TS% demonstrates how much iron is in transit to bone marrow and the liver. TS% is of special value for patients who have been bled too aggressively and whose ferritin stores were depleted too severely. When TS% is high but ferritin is low or low-normal and phlebotomy causes the TS% to rise even more, the patient experiences a condition called iron avidity. This condition is not fully understood, but likely iron avidity is the body's way of assuring survival when iron stores are too low. People who are iron avid are at increased risk for certain infections and should take steps to bring iron back in balance.

How is iron avidity corrected? At the National Institutes of Health, hemochromatosis patients who are iron avid are given iron supplements. At Iron Disorders Institute we recommend first increasing red meat consumption. Meat contains nutrients such as B^{12} and zinc, which are important to blood cell production. Iron pills will replenish iron stores faster, but there may be side effects, such as intestinal upset. Whichever approach is used, it will be up to the individual and his or her physician because either of these approaches, providing there is no other problem present, will bring iron stores back into balance eventually, which is the goal. Discontinuing phlebotomy until the ferritin is over 50 ng/mL (preferably >75ng/mL) is recommended for the iron avid patient, because serum ferritin will drop about 30 ng/mL with each full unit of blood removed.

How do humans regulate absorption of iron? Humans with normal metabolism have the ability to regulate absorption of nutrients such as iron. In times of high need for iron, such as pregnancy, rapid growth and development, or blood loss, the body adjusts to take in more iron. When iron stores are sufficient, the body reduces the amount of iron absorbed from the diet. Some people do not have the benefit of this natural iron regulatory mechanism. People with inherited disorders of iron metabolism such as hemochromatosis have faulty iron regulation and management because of changes in their genes. Of those with iron overload, about 80 percent have two mutated copies of the hemochromatosis gene HFE. Others at risk for iron overload are people with sideroblastic anemia, thalassemia, sickle-cell disease, enzyme deficiencies, and those who are transfusion dependent. With the discovery of other iron regulatory proteins such as hepcidin, ferroportin, transferrin receptors, new gene mutations and new genes, we gain a broader understanding of how non-heme iron is regulated in the human body. More research is needed to learn about heme iron regulation and how diet and behavior impact the iron levels for people with hemochromatosis and other iron-loading disorders.

The Iron Withholding Defense System
Because nature knows that too much iron is harmful, an elaborate and complex system exists in the body to manage iron. Take, for example, the iron withholding defense system which is demonstrated when inflammation is present in the body, a condition that looks like iron deficiency anemia but is in fact a transient condition of defense that provides protection against nourishing harmful pathogens such as cancer cells or bacteria.

Anemia of chronic disease (ACD) is a common condition that can fool a physician into diagnosing iron deficiency anemia (IDA) and recommending iron supplementation. Most patients upon being told they are "anemic" purchase over-the-counter iron and self medicate when, in fact, many of these people are actually exhibiting a "fake anemia;" their natural defense mechanism, called the iron withholding defense system—identified in the late 1970s by Indiana University, Professor of Microbiology, Dr. Eugene Weinberg—has been activated. In an attempt to withhold excess iron from harmful pathogens such as cancer cells or bacteria, the iron withholding defense system is activated in humans whenever an infection, inflammation, or early stages of tumor development are present. Individuals with anemia of chronic disease can experience a slight drop in hemoglobin, low TS% but elevated serum ferritin. This type anemia corrects itself when the underlying disease such as infection, inflammation, or tumor is treated and no longer present. Anyone diagnosed with anemia should also have serum ferritin measured to be certain the anemia is caused by an iron deficiency and not inflammation.

What infections are most dangerous to a person with hemochromatosis? When body iron is in excess, any infection can be dangerous. One in particular is a fairly common bacterium, *Vibrio vulnificus*, which is not harmful to people with normal iron levels, can be deadly to a person with excess tissue iron. Exposure to this bacterium, which is found in raw shellfish such as oysters, has caused deaths of persons with high iron levels.

How is tissue iron lowered? For people with normal hemoglobin levels blood donation or therapeutic phlebotomy is used to reduce iron levels in ferritin. For those with sub-normal hemoglobin values, iron chelation therapy is currently the only way to safely and efficiently remove excess iron. Iron chelation with EDTA is not the same as iron chelation with a prescribed agent that is highly specific for iron, such as deferoxamine (brand Desferal®) and deferasirox (brand Exjade®), both of which are approved for use in the United States; the latter is an oral iron chelator. Deferiprone (brand Ferriprox™) is another oral chelator, but is not yet approved for use in the United States.

What are the types of iron we consume? Humans consume two types of iron: heme iron and nonheme iron.

Heme iron is derived from organic sources such as the blood proteins, hemoglobin, and myoglobin contained in meat. This type of iron is in a form more easily absorbed by the body. About 10 percent or less of dietary iron consumed in American diets is heme iron, even though meat consumption in the US is high. For persons with normal iron metabolism only 20 to 25 percent of the heme iron consumed is actually absorbed. For example, a four-ounce hamburger contains about 3 milligrams of iron; about 1.2 milligrams are heme and about 1.8 milligrams are nonheme. The

> ## WARNING
>
> Persons with iron-loading conditions should not eat raw shellfish and should not walk barefoot on beaches. Some shellfish, such as oysters, contain *Vibrio vulnificus*, a bacterium that can be fatal to persons with high iron levels.

Reprinted with permission from Iron Disorders Institute, 2000

IRON per 3.2 oz serving **MEAT**

	total iron MILLIGRAMS	heme iron percentage of total iron	heme iron MILLIGRAMS
VENISON	4.5	51	2.3
LAMB	3.1	55	1.7
BEEF			
RUMP STEAK	2.9	52	1.5
SIRLOIN STEAK	2.5	52	1.3
ROUND STEAK	3.2	50	1.6
TOP ROUND	2.5	48	1.2
GROUND	2.5	40	1.0
BRISKET	2.0	25	0.5
VEAL	1.9	40*	0.7*
PORK	1.3	23	0.3
PROCESSED MEATS			
SAUSAGE (VEAL)	0.7	40*	0.2*
BOILED HAM	0.7	40*	0.2*
LIVER PATE	5.0	16	0.8
CHICKEN	0.6	40*	0.2*
FISH			
COD	0.2	0.0	0.0
MACKEREL	0.7	0.0	0.0
SALMON	0.6	17	0.1
MUSSELS	4.6	48	2.2
LOBSTER	1.6	40*	0.6*
SHRIMP	2.6	40*	1.0*

* resources vary

amount of heme iron absorbed from that 4-oz. hamburger would be approximately a third of a milligram. People with hereditary hemochromatosis can absorb up to four times the iron of a person with normal iron metabolism. Therefore, 80 to 100 percent of heme iron can be absorbed, or approximately 1.2 milligrams from the same 4-oz. hamburger. Calcium is the only substance that has been found to inhibit heme iron absorption, whereas numerous substances can inhibit the absorption of nonheme iron. Though there are many foods and supplements that will impede or enhance absorption of nonheme iron, absorption of heme iron is little affected by these foods or products.

About 40 to 45 percent of the iron contained in meat is heme, the other 55 to 60 percent is nonheme iron. Iron contained in plants is almost entirely nonheme iron, though plants can contain minute traces of heme iron. Nonheme iron represents the majority of dietary iron humans consume. Nonheme iron is derived from grains, nuts, fruits, vegetables, fortificants, supplements, or contaminant iron such as that derived from water, soil, or cooking utensils. Unlike heme iron, the iron from all these sources must be changed before absorption can take place.

What changes iron so that it can be absorbed? When nonheme iron is ingested it is in a form called ferric iron. Ferric iron cannot be absorbed by humans; when ferric iron reaches the stomach, it mixes with stomach acid (hydrochloric acid) and is changed into ferrous iron. Ferrous iron is the form of iron that can be absorbed; it moves out of the stomach into the first part of the intestine called the duodenum. This is the point at which scientists believe the majority of absorption takes place. Some scientists speculate that there is another absorption site farther down in the intestinal tract where minute amounts of iron can absorbed, but this theory is still being researched.

Can diet reduce stored iron levels? Not for a person with serious iron overload; only blood loss or reduced red blood cell production will efficiently lower iron levels. A dietary plan can significantly reduce absorption of iron from the diet and therefore reduce the amount of iron sent to storage in ferritin. Reduced absorption can lower the number of therapeutic phlebotomies needed for many with hemochromatosis-related iron overload. One can induce iron deficiency anemia with a specialized diet, such as a strict vegetarian diet. Also, taking a daily aspirin and vigorous exercise can cause minute amounts of intestinal blood loss. These measures can contribute to tissue iron reduction but are considered preventive measures more than therapeutic approaches.

Is there a pill that will reduce iron levels? Yes. Deferasirox (Exjade®) is available in the United States, but is not yet approved for use by persons with hemochromatosis. When a drug is not approved for a specific use but a physician prescribes it anyway, use of the drug is called "off-label" and the patient may have to pay for it out of pocket. Another pill, deferiprone (Ferriprox®) is on the market but not approved for use in the United States. Iron Disorders Institute does not recommend iron chelator pills in place of phlebotomy for people who can tolerate blood removal. One phlebotomy takes about twenty minutes and removes about 250 milligrams of iron! Iron chelators require daily drug administration to remove about two-thirds the iron that a full phlebotomy will remove in a month: in other words, phlebotomy removes ~1,000 mgs compared to the ~650 mgs removed by the chelator method. Hemochromatosis patients who cannot tolerate phlebotomy for whatever reason are candidates for iron chelation with these drugs because lower excess levels of iron is crucial to survival. However, as long as a hemochromatosis patient's hemoglobin remains sufficient for phlebotomy or blood donation, this method is the recommended way to remove excess tissue iron.

What is the best diet plan for someone with hemochromatosis? No single food or substance is a cure-all; balance is the key. A good diet plan for anyone, including someone with an iron imbalance, needs to be simple and incorporate all food groups. It also needs to be easy to follow and adhere to, and it needs to be dynamic and changing, as the individual's needs change. All foods, including those rich in vitamin C, should remain in the diet of a person with hemochromatosis. *The Hemochromatosis Cookbook* teaches a person simple techniques that allow for all foods with the exception of organ meats, raw shellfish, and animal fat to be consumed.

Every person is different. A person with iron overload doesn't fit neatly into a single patient profile. Some people have elevated serum ferritin with only slightly elevated saturation percentages. These individuals may need only a few phlebotomies and minor dietary changes. Some people have extremely high iron levels and need long-term, aggressive phlebotomy. Some are smokers and some consume excessive amounts of alcohol, two behaviors that amplify risk of disease, especially in the presence of excessive iron. These individuals might need a strict diet and an aggressive therapeutic phlebotomy regimen. Others may be totally deironed and just want to maintain healthy iron levels by controlling absorption of the metal. Recipes in *The Hemochromatosis Cookbook* were first published in *Cooking with Less Iron* and remain the favorites of people who aim to cook with less iron. Some of the recipes have been altered slightly for improved flavor or for the prediabetic or diabetic hemochromatosis patient. All recipes are still helpful for balancing iron while enjoying favorite foods such as beef, venison, eggs, and spinach. People just diagnosed and who have very high tissue iron levels may want to plan the majority of their meals from this book and follow the eating plan closely. Persons who are deironed and want to minimize the amount of iron absorbed might select recipes from this book two or three times a week.

The Hemochromatosis Cookbook eating plan allows for flexibility with its suggested substitutions and provides for reward meals, such as a beef entrée periodically. With the exception of reduction of some harmful substances or supplemental iron, no nutrient or food group is eliminated from the daily diet. Measures to reduce the amount of iron absorbed are incorporated into the eating plan. Recipes in this book were taste-tested and selected for their universal appeal.

What about supplementation? A daily iron-free multivitamin is recommended, especially for patients undergoing phlebotomy. Phlebotomy removes nutrients other than iron, such as zinc and copper. Taking a daily multivitamin is one way to replenish nutrients lost during phlebotomy. Avoid supplements that require a dosage of 6 to 8 pills a day. In addition to being expensive, taking high doses of supplements may also cause gastrointestinal discomfort or undue stress on the liver. When selecting a daily vitamin, choose a "one-dose" pill with vitamin A content of less than 4,500 IU. High doses of vitamin A can cause liver failure.

Bioavailability of iron

In recent decades scientists have found ways that are more sensitive in detecting the effects of substances on the absorption of iron, including nutrients such as beta carotene, zinc, copper, and calcium. Dr. Raymond Glahn of the Cornell University Agricultural Research Division of the USDA developed an artificial gut that provides for better accuracy in establishing bioavailability of iron from the diet. "Bioavailability" is the extent to which a nutrient or drug is accessible to the body for its intended use. According to Dr. Janet Hunt of the Agricultural Research Team, Grand Forks Human Nutrition Research Center, "Iron absorption from food can vary up to ten-fold, depending on the bioavailability of iron." Prior to modern inventions such as the artificial gut and breakthroughs in genetics, scientists had few methods for determining iron absorption with such precision. Dr. Miguel Layrisse, a world-renowned expert in absorption, provides a brief description of how science has studied absorption.

Absorption of iron

In the '40s iron absorption was determined by chemistry. The amount of iron absorbed was calculated as the difference between dietary iron and excreted iron. The other method used to measure dietary iron was hemoglobin repletion. In the '70s the measurement of plasma ferritin was an important contribution to iron metabolism to assess iron deficiency and iron overload. In the same decade the extrinsic and intrinsic labeled methodology was an important advancement. The '70s and '80s were years where scientists aimed at finding iron absorption inhibitors, namely coffee, calcium, tea, zinc and fiber. The '80s and '90s were characterized for the emerging knowledge of iron absorption from a food, a meal, and a complete diet and for the favorable effect of food iron fortification in developing countries. Also the effect of iron excess in overall health and myocardial infarction in developed countries was studied.

—Dr. Miguel Layrisse, Centro de Medicina Experimental, Instituto Venezolano de Investigaciones Cientificas Center for Experimental Medicine and Institute for Scientific Investigations, University of Central Venezuela

What foods increase or inhibit absorption of iron?
Substances that increase iron absorption: *Ascorbic acid,* or Vitamin C, occurs naturally in vegetables and fruits, especially citrus; it can also be synthesized for use in supplements. Ascorbic acid enhances the absorption of nutrients such as iron. One glass of orange juice (about 100 milligrams (mg) of vitamin C) can counteract the iron-inhibiting effect of a cup of tea. Studies suggest that greater than or equal to 50 mg of ascorbic acid would be required to overcome the inhibitory effects on iron absorption of any meal containing greater than 100 mg of tannic acid contained in coffee, tea, and some foods, such as grapes, red rices, or eggplant. In studies concerning the effects of ascorbic acid on iron absorption, 100 mg of ascorbic acid increased iron absorption from a specific meal by 4.14 times. In a standard meal of meat, potatoes, and milk, 100 mg of ascorbic acid increased absorption of iron by 67 percent. The addition of 100 mg of ascorbic acid to a specially formulated liquid meal containing 85 mg of phytate increased absorption by 3.14 times. Naturally occurring vitamin C in fruits and vegetables should not be restricted from the diet. However, supplemental vitamin C—ascorbic acid—should be restricted to less than 200 mg per dose and should not be taken with high-iron meals.

Alcohol enhances iron absorption. Light to moderate consumption of alcohol has known health benefits, but heavy or abusive drinking, especially when

ABSORPTION OF IRON
foods & substances that *increase* absorption
ascorbic acid (vitamin C)
alcohol
beta-carotene
meat, some fish
EDTA +Fe
Ferrochel®
hydrochloric acid
sugar
drugs (nicotine)
foods & substances that *reduce* absorption
polyphenols and phenols tannins (tea, coffee) chlorogenic acid (chocolate) phenolic acid (apples)
oxalates (oregano, spinach)
eggs
phytates (fiber)
phosphates in dairy
calcium
sources: see bibliography

Reprinted with permission from Iron Disorders Institute, 2007 in combination with high body iron levels, increases the risk for liver damage and liver cancer. Studies show that heavy drinkers have high iron levels. Approximately 20 to 30 percent of those who are heavy consumers of alcohol acquire up to twice the amount of dietary iron as do moderate or light drinkers. Alcohol will hasten liver disease, such as cirrhosis. Patients who have developed cirrhosis increase their chance of developing liver cancer by up to 200-fold. Alcohol in the presence of high iron can also cause brain damage. Alcohol-induced lab rats were found to have an alarming amount of "free iron" in the cells of their brains. A "standard drink" is defined as 13.5 grams of alcohol, or: 12 ounces of beer, 5 ounces of wine, 1.5 ounces of distilled spirits. "Moderate consumption" is defined as two drinks per day for an adult male; one drink per day for females or those older than 65 regardless of gender. Options to consider might be nonalcoholic or low-alcohol-content beer and wine. Though red wine is reported to be healthy for the heart, it is likely the polyphenol content in red wine that is providing the greater benefit. Except for the sedating quality of alcohol, a handful of red grapes will provide equal, if not greater, health benefit.

> **WARNING**
>
> Grapefruit juice can cause serious side effects, including fatalities, when taken with certain medications. Something in the fruit causes drug potency to be increased up to twelve-fold.

Beta-carotene is one of more than 100 carotenoids that occur naturally in plants and animals. Carotenoids are yellow to red pigments that are contained in foods such as apricots, beets and beet greens, carrots, collard greens, corn, red grapes, oranges, peaches, prunes, red peppers, spinach, sweet potatoes, tomatoes, turnip greens, and yellow squash. Beta-carotene enables the body to produce vitamin A. In studies of the effects of vitamin A and beta-carotene on absorption of iron, vitamin A

FOODS HIGH IN BETA-CAROTENE
micrograms/100 grams edible portion

Food	Amount
Apricots	2,554
Asparagus	493
Beets	2,560
Broccoli	1,042
Brussels sprouts	465
Butter with salt	158
Carrots	8,836
Chard	3,954
Cilantro	3,440
Collards	4,418
Endive	960
Grape leaves (canned)	2,838
Grapefruit (pink)	603
Kale (cooked)	6,202
Lettuce (Romaine)	1,272
Lettuce (iceberg)	192
Mangos (fresh)	445
Margarine spread	721
Melon (cantaloupe)	1,595
Okra	170
Orange (fresh)	122
Papayas (fresh)	276
Peaches (fresh)	97
Peas	320
Peppers green	22
Peppers red	2,220
Peppers yellow	120
Spinach (cooked)	5,242
Spinach (raw)	5,597
Squash (yellow)	90
Squash (zucchini)	410
Sweet potato	9,488
Tomatoes (paste)	1,242
Tomatoes fresh	393

Beta-Carotene is one of the carotenoids, which are the red, green, yellow and orange pigments found in fruits and vegetables. Beta-Carotene enables the body to produce vitamin A and is highly effective as an antioxidant.

This important nutrient should not be eliminated from the diet because of the health benefits it provides.

did not significantly increase iron absorption under the experimental conditions employed. However, beta-carotene significantly increased absorption of the metal. Moreover, in the presence of phytates or tannic acid, beta-carotene generally overcame the inhibitory effects of both compounds, depending on their concentrations. Like vitamin E, beta-carotene is an excellent anti-oxidant; naturally occurring beta-carotene or vitamin E in foods should not be restricted from the diet.

EDTA+fe and *Ferrochel*™ are additive iron compounds and are emerging as the fortifiers of choice by major food manufacturers. Individuals with conditions such as hemochromatosis who are at high risk for iron overload will need to avoid food products fortified with these two compounds. Both additives were found to exceed absorption capabilities of the commonly used fortifier ferrous sulfate.

Ferrochel™ is an iron bis-glycine chelate. Glycine is a nonessential amino acid used as a chelate. This chelate has a 2:1 ratio to the mineral, hence, "bis" meaning "two" glycines to one iron atom. Albion Laboratories, Salt Lake City, Utah, owns the patent rights to produce this type of chelate, which is much more effective at delivering a high bioavailable form of iron than ferrous sulfate.

Fe-EDTA is a compound of iron salts and EDTA (ethylenediaminetetra-acetic acid), a broad-spectrum chelate, which means it binds with many minerals. It too performed well in the same absorption studies. Both EDTA and bis-glycine-chelated iron were absorbed at the rate of two to three times that of ferrous sulfate. When combined with phytase, the enzyme that breaks down phytates in fiber, Ferrochel™ and EDTA increase the bioavailability of iron even more.

Hydrochloric acid is the acid found in the stomach that breaks down food and makes it available for absorption. Antacids, proton pump inhibitors, and calcium supplements can reduce the amount of hydrochloric acid in the stomach. Taking these inhibiting compounds is not recommended for persons with iron-loading conditions.

Meat, especially red meat, increases the absorption of nonheme iron. Beef, lamb, and venison contain the highest amounts of heme, as compared to pork or chicken, which contain low amounts of heme. Meat also contains animal fats, which can increase absorption of nonheme iron. It has been calculated that 1 gram of meat (about 20 percent protein) has an enhancing effect on nonheme iron absorption equivalent to that of 1 milligram of ascorbic acid. A Latin American–type meal (maize, rice, and black beans) with a low iron bioavailability had the same improved bioavailability when either 75 g of meat or 50 mg of ascorbic acid were added. Fats (lipids) and iron are a perfect combination for free-radical activity and cell death.

Sugar

Researchers investigated the absorption rates of seven different beverages that contained sugar and were fortified with iron. They found that sugar improved the absorption of iron by as much as four times in some cases. Since this study, others have determined that the risk of developing high iron stores in subjects who consumed more than twenty-one servings of high-sugar fruits or fruit juice per week was three-fold more than in the subjects who consumed fourteen servings per week.

Drugs

Products that contain nicotine, such as tobacco or stop-smoking gums, will increase iron absorption.

Substances That Inhibit Absorption of Iron

Polyphenols are phenolic compounds, such as chlorogenic acid found in cocoa, coffee, and some herbs. Phenolic acid found in apples, peppermint, and some herbal teas, and tannins found in black teas, coffee, cocoa, spices, walnuts, and fruits such as apples, blackberries, raspberries, and blueberries all contain polyphenols. Of the polyphenols, Swedish cocoa and certain teas demonstrate the most powerful iron-absorption-inhibiting capabilities, in some cases up to 90 percent. Coffee is high in tannin and chlorogenic acid; one cup of certain types of coffee can inhibit iron absorption by as much as 60 percent. *Tannin warning:* Excessive consumption of tannin is not recommended for people with liver damage or disease. One glass of tea, a cup of coffee, or small amount of red wine with a meal will probably be allowed, but talk with your doctor about the condition of your liver and the consumption of tannins.

Phytate is a compound contained in soy protein and fiber found in walnuts, almonds, sesame seeds, dried beans, lentils and peas, cereals, and whole grains. Recent absorption studies in humans have demonstrated that even low levels of phytate (about 5 percent of the amounts in cereal whole flours) have a strong inhibitory effect on iron absorption. Phytate levels are reduced during yeast fermentation in rye, white, and whole wheat breads, and sourdough leavening results in an almost complete degradation of phytate.

Phosphates are compounds used to whiten food products; they are found in modified tapioca starch, bacon, toothpaste, certain medications, and some dairy products. The ability of phosphates to inhibit the absorption of iron is not completely understood.

Calcium is an essential mineral; it is found in foods such as milk, yogurt, cheese, sardines, canned salmon, tofu, broccoli, almonds, figs, turnip greens, and rhubarb.

Reports that calcium can impair the absorption of both heme and nonheme iron have been supported by the USDA Agricultural Research Department. Where 50 milligrams or less of calcium had no effect on absorption, calcium in amounts 300 to 600 milligrams inhibited the absorption of heme iron similarly to nonheme iron. One cup of skim milk contains about 300 milligrams of calcium.

Oxalates are compounds derived from oxalic acid and are found in foods such as spinach, kale, beets, nuts, chocolate, tea, wheat bran, rhubarb, strawberries, and herbs such as oregano, basil, and parsley. Oxalates impair the absorption of nonheme iron. The presence of oxalates in spinach explains why the iron in spinach is not absorbed. In fact, it is reported that the iron from spinach that does get absorbed is probably from the minute particles of sand or dirt clinging to the plant rather than the iron contained in the plant itself.

Eggs are often mistakenly removed from the diet because of the high iron content of the egg yolk. Eggs actually work to impair absorption of iron because of a phosphoprotein called phosvitin. The binding capacity of this protein with iron may be responsible for the low bioavailability of iron from eggs and possibly the iron-inhibiting ability of eggs called the "egg factor." The egg factor has been observed in several separate studies. One boiled egg can reduce absorption of iron in a meal by as much as 28 percent.

Zinc is an essential mineral found in meat, eggs, seafood, and to some degree in grains. High doses of supplemental zinc can interfere with copper utilization, which can lead to impaired metabolism of iron.

Fats can increase iron absorption to some degree, but more important, some fats are oxidized by iron, which triggers free-radical production and results in cell death.

Fats—Good and Bad

When we think of fat, images of oozing butter, greasy potato chips, and thick, juicy steaks might come to mind. Fat-free diets continue to be followed faithfully by people still under the false impression that all fat is bad. Recent research indicates that certain fats actually lower the bad type of cholesterol, reduce triglycerides, and lower blood pressure.

Fats, also called fatty acids, include *saturated* and *unsaturated* fats:

- Saturated fats are derived from both plant and animal sources and have been shown to promote plaque formation by raising blood cholesterol in animals and humans. Saturated fats are solid at room temperature. Those derived from animal sources include fat contained in the flesh of meat or products such as bacon, lard, butter, whole milk, cream, ice cream, and cheese. Saturated fats can contribute to clogged arteries as well as elevated bad cholesterol, triglycerides, and blood pressure.

- Trans-unsaturated fats are formed from a chemical process know as hydrogenation, where a liquid fat is made into a solid by the process of adding hydrogen atoms to an unsaturated fat. Consumption of trans fats has been shown to increase the risk of heart disease. Hydrogenation gives foods, such as crackers, cookies, potato chips, French fries, and doughnuts, a longer shelf-life by making them less likely to turn rancid. Only recently have food manufacturers begun to label products with the type of fats used; while some manufacturers are completely eliminating trans fats from their products, the food often still contains high fats.

Saturated and trans-unsaturated fats can be catalysts for chemical reactions in the body that can cause free-radical activity. Free radicals contribute to degenerative disease and hasten the aging process. Iron can provide the oxygen fat needs to set off this chemical reaction. A rotting apple or the rust on an automobile is an example of oxygen + iron free-radical activity. Eat these types of fat sparingly.

Unsaturated fats are liquid at room temperature. There are two types of unsaturated fats: polyunsaturated and monounsaturated. Within the polyunsaturated fats are yet another two types: Omega-6 and Omega-3 polyunsaturated fatty acids. One can be harmful to health; the other beneficial.

Polyunsaturated fatty acids (PUFA): Omega-6 PUFA are derived from vegetable oils and are liquid at room temperature. They include corn, sunflower, safflower, soybean, and sesame oils. Salad dressing, margarine, and mayonnaise containing these oils are therefore are high in polyunsaturated fat; eat these sparingly.

Omega-3 PUFA, found primarily in fish, is a good type of polyunsaturated fat. Omega-3 polyunsaturated fats do not increase serum cholesterol or LDL levels. Their effects are shown to lower the risk of cardiovascular disease and breast cancer. For persons concerned about iron in fish, the type of iron in most fish is primarily nonheme iron. Certain food substances, such as tannin, fiber, and dairy, can inhibit the absorption of this type of iron. Fish, therefore, is an excellent protein choice and should be included in one's diet at least three to four times a week. Coldwater fish are among the best choices. One German study reported that omega-3 fatty acids may decrease malignant metastatic tumor growth in the liver.

Other Good Fats

Monounsaturated fats are derived from plant sources. High amounts are found in olive, canola (rapeseed), and peanut oil, as well as avocados and certain nuts. Monounsaturated fats do not increase serum cholesterol or LDL levels. Their effects are shown to lower the risk of cardiovascular disease and breast cancer because these oils may contribute to lowering cholesterol levels.

We need fats in our diet for normal metabolism and body function. A healthy diet is low in animal fats and hydrogenated fats but includes good fats such as olive oil and those found in coldwater fish.

Hemochromatosis Eating Plan

Humans need nutrients such as fats, carbohydrates, protein, vitamins, minerals including iron, and adequate amounts of water to assure proper metabolism and optimal health. All foods contain some nutrients the body can utilize. Choosing the best source of a nutrient and eating these foods in balance and moderation is the key to enjoying a wide variety of tastes, including desserts. With the exception of foods to which one is allergic or foods restricted because of diabetes or other sensitivities, a hemochromatosis patient can modify his or her diet and incorporate nearly all foods.

When tissue iron levels are very high, hemochromatosis patients will want to be more restrictive with their diet. In these cases, the patients should reduce the amount of heme iron consumed and incorporate foods that impede absorption of nonheme iron. People with HHC have the ability to absorb quadruple the iron that a person with normal metabolism absorbs. These people still need iron for body function; they just need less of it.

HEMOCHROMATOSIS EATING PLAN CHECKLIST

! ■ **IMPORTANT! The following suggested diet restrictions are for patients with very high iron levels. Once a person achieves iron balance, some of these approaches can result in iron deficiency anemia.**

1. Plan ahead.
2. Note the nonheme and heme iron content in foods.
3. Incorporate foods and substances that limit absorption of iron.
4. Do not eat raw shellfish.
5. Include low-sugar fresh fruits and non-starchy & leafy green vegetables.
6. Limit supplemental vitamin C to 200 milligrams.
7. Limit alcohol; avoid if liver damage is present.
8. Take a daily multivitamin.
9. Include good fats.
10. Limit use of iron skillets.
11. Limit nicotine.
12. Get plenty of fluids.
13. Stick to a phlebotomy schedule.

Reprinted with permission from Iron Disorders Institute, 2000

The Hemochromatosis Cookbook eating plan is formulated for persons with conditions of iron overload such as hereditary hemochromatosis. Recipes are balanced for the majority of persons who incorporate some physical activity into their daily routine and do not smoke or drink excessively.

Any eating plan must be adjusted to meet the individual needs of persons with chronic conditions. Persons with arthritis, diabetes, heart disease, liver disease, cancer, and who are overweight or in chronic pain will want to adjust recipes for best results.

Variety is key; any food might be tolerated occasionally but "occasionally" must be defined. For some, the word *occasionally* might mean every three days, once a week, once a month, etc. Discuss diet with a nutritionist to determine how often exceptions to a prescribed diet may occur.

Everyone is different; not all hemochromatosis patients have the same iron levels, eat the same foods, or have the same habits. Patients with very high iron levels: serum ferritin over 1,000 ng/mL will need to take greater precautions. Once iron levels are lowered to a serum ferritin under 1,000 ng/mL, some liberties can be taken. But it is important to point out that iron reduction therapy must continue until the body iron levels are within normal range.

MYTH: *Spinach, eggs and red meat are high in iron and should be eliminated from the diet of people with hemochromatosis.*

Although red meat contains the most absorbable form of iron (heme iron), *The Hemochromatosis Cookbook* teaches you how to enjoy red meat (lamb, venison, or beef) in a way that reduces the amount of iron absorbed. Spinach contains a compound that actually impairs the absorption of iron; so do eggs. See why you need not remove these foods from the diet.

Once iron levels are within normal range, providing there is no liver damage or other metabolic abnormality, the hemochromatosis patient can resume eating red meat, consume alcohol in moderation, and may not need to intake tannins or calcium in order to control iron absorption. If, however, the patient is iron avid, raw shellfish must be avoided and an added precaution must be taken against exposure to infection.

Thirteen Steps to a Healthy Eating Plan

1. *Plan ahead.*

   Deciding what meals will be consumed during a week helps save money and reduces the number of impulsive decisions to eat what is handy. Often these choices are fast food or foods that are not nutritious. Planning ahead offers opportunities for reward meals such as an occasional lean cut of steak or glass of red wine. Use the blank menu planner on page 43, referring to the sample week of menus as a guideline. Leave the shopping list in a convenient place so that as certain foods are depleted they can be noted for the next trip to the grocery store.

2. *With the menu planner, calculate the nonheme and heme iron content in foods.*
   Use the food composition charts and the blank worksheets provided in this book to calculate the amount of iron in foods you intend to incorporate into your weekly meal plan. Visit www.hemochromatosis.org or www.irondisorders.org and click on the links for diet and iron content in foods. Also, see the section on Food Values to help determine protein, carbohydrate, and fat content of foods.

3. *Incorporate foods and substances that impair absorption of iron: tea, coffee, dairy, fiber.*

4. *Do not eat raw shellfish and take precaution when walking barefooted on beaches.*
   Oysters especially can be contaminated with *Vibrio vulnificus*; when consumed by a person with high iron, the result may be death by septicemia if emergency medical attention is not received. Usually, IV antibiotic is the emergency treatment.

5. *Eat freely of low-sugar fruits and high-fiber vegetables (unless you are diabetic):*
   Fruits such as berries, apples, and kiwi versus ripe or high-sugar fruits are the best choices when iron levels are high. Berries are also good fruit choices for diabetics. Eventually you can begin to mix in some of the riper, higher-sugar-content fruits (e.g., bananas, pineapple) once iron levels are closer to normal. Do not be concerned about vitamin C or beta-carotene content of these antioxidant-rich foods. Potatoes when eaten with the skins, for example, are very high in fiber. The iron content is not likely to be absorbed.

6. *Limit supplemental vitamin C to 200 milligrams per dose.*

7. *Limit the amount of alcohol consumed with the meal.*

8. *Take a daily iron-free vitamin supplement.*

9. *Consume good fats:*
   Use olive oil for cooking and salad dressings. Enjoy raw avocados and coconuts, which are rich in nutrients and fats known to lower the risk of some cancers.

10. *Avoid cooking in cast-iron skillets or on grills.*
    Cook in glassware when possible, but you do not have to a fanatic about it. Cornbread cooked in an iron skillet is a real treat that should not be lost to someone with hemochromatosis. The real issue with the cast-iron skillet is to not let foods simmer for long periods or eat high-acid foods (e.g., tomatoes)

cooked in an iron skillet. Once iron levels are back down to normal, there is no reason not to enjoy an occasional iron skillet meal.

11. *Be compliant with iron reduction therapy (i.e., phlebotomy, medication).*
    No diet can replace this important aspect of therapy for those with iron overload.

12. *Keep hydrated.*
    Your body can get some water from foods, but most people tend not to eat adequate amounts of foods with high water content, such as fruits and vegetables. Investigators have demonstrated that a sodium-coconut water mixture hydrates as well as sports drinks and with better fluid tolerance. Adequate hydration reduces the time it takes to remove a pint of blood.

13. *Don't smoke, chew tobacco, and limit nicotine consumption.*

Hemochromatosis Diabetes*

Diabetes mellitus is a common consequence for people with hemochromatosis. More than 90 percent of hemochromatosis patients with diabetes have Type II diabetes or are glucose intolerant, and about one-third of these patients require insulin.

Iron can cause damage to tissues of vital organs by changing oxygen into a form known as free radical–increased oxidative stress. Unopposed free-radical activity can cause irreversible cell damage. It is believed that this is how iron destroys the beta cells, causing diabetes. Beta cells or islet cells have very low levels of the enzymes that break down free radicals. Thus, agents that increase free-radical production, such as iron, could result in destruction of pancreatic cells.

Iron reduction for the majority of hemochromatosis patients is therapeutic phlebotomy or periodic blood donation. This is the safest, most cost effective way to lower excessive body iron stores. If the patient has anemia, phlebotomy may be accompanied by or replaced with other therapeutic approaches using pharmaceuticals such as iron chelators or erythropoietin.

Some hemochromatosis patients with diabetes have reported that when iron levels were returned to normal range, insulin- or glucose-control medication was no longer needed. Everyone is different, and not everyone can follow the exact same approach for disease management. No one should discontinue medication without medical advice and supervision; you and your physician will determine what is best in your situation.

Hemochromatosis patients with diabetes can follow the same diet guidelines as a person with diabetes who does not have hemochromatosis. The hemochromatosis eating plan checklist can be added to recipes for diabetics, as there are no known problems for diabetics having coffee or tea, which contain tannins. Decaffeinated teas and coffees are recommended for diabetics.

Common sense good-health practices, such as regular physical activity, reducing consumption of animal fats, white sugar, and processed foods, reducing alcohol consumption and quitting the use of tobacco and nicotine, are fundamental to any sensible diet plan. To this list we add maintaining iron balance, a practice that is not limited to patients with hemochromatosis. Iron balance is vital to good health for any age, gender, or ethnicity.

---

*This chapter is an excerpt from Iron Disorders Institute newsletter nanograms 2nd Quarter 2008 and is reprinted with permission.

As stated earlier, treatment for a hemochromatosis patient with high iron levels is therapeutic phlebotomy. Frequency and the amount of blood removed are critical to iron balance. A patient may need multiple phlebotomies a week or only a few a year. A common problem for hemochromatosis patients is overbleeding, which often results in a condition called iron avidity. Iron avidity is when the serum ferritin is below normal but the transferrin-iron saturation percentage is high; the hemoglobin is usually normal. For more information on iron avidity see page 19.

The hemochromatosis patient is now an iron-deficient patient. Many physicians continue to order phlebotomies, in some cases partial phlebotomies in an attempt to bring down the TS%. In fact, the TS% is probably a consequence of chronic blood loss.

Bringing iron levels back into balance for the iron avid hemochromatosis patient requires measures that would be unthinkable in the past. Discontinuing phlebotomies, taking iron pills, and eating red meat become part of the routine to get iron levels back up to normal. This can pose a challenge for diabetic patients who generally are not allowed much red meat.

The Iron Disorders Institute provides information about iron balance control; this information is on IDI's websites (irondisorders.org and hemochromatosis.org). There are many resources for information on diabetes control. Talk with your nutritionist or healthcare provider about literature and resources. We recommend visiting the National Diabetes Clearinghouse website: http://diabetes.niddk.nih.gov/dm/pubs/overview/index.htm. From this site you can find countless resources, such as links, literature, articles, clinical trials, statistics, definitions, therapies, and prevention programs.

If you are a hemochromatosis patient with diabetes, the Iron Disorders Institute recommends that you:
1. Consult with a healthcare provider to determine the best therapeutic approach for blood sugar control and the best physical activity program.
2. Consult with a diabetes nutrition specialist to discuss portion control, eating schedules, and supplements.
3. Work out menus in advance.
4. Determine the amount of heme and nonheme iron in a meal.
5. Determine the calorie, protein, fat, and carbohydrate content of a meal.
6. Discuss the menu selections with a nutritionist.
7. Have regular consultations and checkups for blood work to assure good blood sugar, iron, and weight control.
8. Use evidence-based resources.

Portion control is a vital part of any diet plan. The following section from the National Institute of Diabetes and Digestive and Kidney Diseases provides calorie intake and portion-size guidelines by gender and stature for diabetic meal planning.

Have about 1,200 to 1,600 calories a day if you are a
- small woman who exercises
- small or medium-sized woman who wants to lose weight
- medium-sized woman who does not exercise much

To have 1,200 to 1,600 calories a day, choose:

6 starches	2 milks
3 vegetables	4 to 6 ounces meat and meat substitutes
2 fruits	up to 3 fats

Have about 1,600 to 2,000 calories a day if you are a
- large woman who wants to lose weight
- small man at a healthy weight
- medium-sized man who does not exercise much
- medium-sized or large man who wants to lose weight

To have 1,600 to 2,000 calories a day, choose:

8 starches	2 milks
4 vegetables	4 to 6 ounces meat and meat substitutes
3 fruits	up to 4 fats

Have about 2,000 to 2,400 calories a day if you are a
- medium-sized or large man who exercises a lot or has a physically active job
- large man at a healthy weight
- medium-sized or large woman who exercises a lot or has a physically active job

To have 2,000 to 2,400 calories a day, choose:

10 starches	2 milks
4 vegetables	5 to 7 ounces meat and meat substitutes
4 fruits	up to 5 fats

Guide to Sensible Serving Sizes

This much	is the same as
	3 ounces 1 serving of meat, chicken, turkey, or fish
	1 cup 1 serving of • cooked vegetables • salads • casseroles or stews, such as chili with beans • milk
	½ cup 1 serving of • fruit or fruit juice • starchy vegetables, such as potatoes or corn • pinto beans and other dried beans • rice or noodles • cereal
	1 ounce 1 serving of • snack food • cheese (1 slice)
	1 tablespoon 1 serving of • salad dressing • cream cheese
	1 teaspoon 1 serving of • margarine or butter • oil

Source: http://diabetes.niddk.nih.gov/dm/pubs/eating_ez/index.htm

Menu Planning and Food Values

Important: The sample menu planners and recipes in The Hemochromatosis Cookbook *are suggestions. Menu planning and changes in diet should be discussed with a healthcare provider and nutritionist, especially for hemochromatosis diabetes patients. Patients with liver disease should limit excessive consumption of tannins, which can be harmful to a liver that is damaged or compromised.*

Some serving sizes appear with recipes
Sauces can be omitted to reduce calories

HEMOCHROMATOSIS SAMPLE MENU PLANNER

	day one	day two	day three	day four	day five	day six	day seven
Breakfast	2 egg western omelet 1/2 cup blueberries red potato homefries coffee	3/4 cup Kellogg brand Complete Oat Bran cereal 1/2 banana (not overripe) 1/2 cup low fat milk coffee	bran muffin with walnuts Neufchatel cheese 1 medium pear coffee	scrambled eggs 1/2 cup seedless grapes Canadian bacon cinnamon toast coffee	frozen yogurt shake 1/4 cup fresh pineapple apple bran muffin coffee	oatmeal with 1/2 banana & faux molasses rye toast coffee	sausage fritatta 1/2 cup blueberries oat bran English muffin coffee
AM snack	V-8 juice daily vitamin	1/2 cantaloupe daily vitamin	1/2 cup peaches daily vitamin	1 medium orange daily vitamin	1/2 grapefruit daily vitamin	1/2 cup fresh strawberries daily vitamin	1 plum daily vitamin
Lunch	minestroni grilled cheese on multigrain bread iced coffee latte	1/2 ham & turkey sub on whole grain with Italian dressing & spicy mustard, 1 cup veggie soup iced tea	pita fajita: chicken, peppers & onions, tomato soup iced tea	pasta fagiole green salad with Italian dressing & herbed croutons iced tea	turkey chili small Caesar's salad with seasoned croutons iced tea	veggie Pocket sandwich with cheddar cheese soup iced tea	1/2 turkey club cream of potato soup iced tea
PM snack optional	1 oz cheese small apple	peanut butter and apple jelly sandwich 1/2 cup lowfat milk	celery sticks with peanut butter apple juice	fresh squeezed lemonade herbed* popcorn	cinnamon toast hot mulled cider	5-6 raw carrot sticks 1 oz peanuts	Hungarian cheese spread with saltine crackers
Dinner	salmon patties with horse radish sauce steamed broccoli macaroni & cheese cornbread tea	barbecued chicken cole slaw Italian cut green beans cornbread tea	oven fried catfish sauteed cabbage & onion, baked beets herb roll tea	ham with mustard sauce broccoli casserole 1/2 baked yam herb bread sticks tea	broiled haddock with herbs steamed asparagus with hollandaise wild rice herb roll tea	marinated flank steak cauliflower cheese sauce steamed okra herbed garlic toast tea	sesame chicken 1/2 twice baked potato steamed spinach tea
Dessert	mocha angel food cake decaf coffee	chocolate cake decaf coffee	carrot cake decaf coffee	banana pudding decaf coffee	chocolate mousse decaf coffee	lime Jell-O salad decaf coffee	sugar cream pie decaf coffee
Before-bed snack	cup of hot Ovaltine made with low fat milk	1/2 cup vanilla yogurt with a pinch of cinnamon	cup of hot Ovaltine made with low fat milk	1/2 cup apple juice 1 oz swiss cheese	1 saltine cracker with peanut butter 1/2 cup cold low fat milk	cup of hot Ovaltine made with low fat milk	1/2 cup vanilla yogurt with a pinch of cinnamon

Remove this page and photocopy at 130% or contact Iron Disorders Institute for enlarged sheet

HEMOCHROMATOSIS MENU PLANNER BLANK

	day one	day two	day three	day four	day five	day six	day seven
Breakfast							
AM snack							
Lunch							
PM snack optional							
Dinner							
Dessert							
Before-bed snack							

Remove this page and photocopy at 130% or contact Iron Disorders Institute for enlarged sheet

HEMOCHROMATOSIS Diabetic SAMPLE MENU PLANNER

Some serving sizes appear with recipes
For guidelines only; discuss with your nutritionist

	day one	day two	day three	day four	day five	day six	day seven
Breakfast	2 egg-white western omelet 1 slice rye crisp 1/4 cup blueberries coffee or tea	3/4 cup Quaker Wheat Puffs cereal 1/4 banana (not overripe) 1/2 cup low-fat cottage cheese coffee or tea	bran muffin with walnuts 1/2 cup low fat cottage cheese 1/2 medium pear coffee or tea	1 scrambled egg with herbs, parmesan cheese & 1 oz lean ham. 1/4 cup seedless grapes coffee or tea	frozen low-fat, yogurt smoothie 1/4 cup fresh berries scoop of sugar-free protein powder coffee or tea	oatmeal with 1/4 cup berries 1 oz of Canadian bacon coffee or tea	turkey sausage fritatta 1/2 cup low fat cottage cheese with apple slices coffee or tea
AM snack daily vitamin	1/8 slice of cantaloupe with 1/4 cup cottage cheese	1/2 cup V-8 juice 1 slice of yogurt cheese	1/ cup fresh strawberries 1 oz of lean ham	1/4 cup fresh raspberries; 1 rye crisp with thin layer of low-fat cream-cheese	1/2 cup V-8 juice 1 slice of yogurt cheese	1/2 pear 2 Tbs. low fat cottage cheese	1/ cup fresh strawberries 1 oz of lean ham
Lunch	Adam Tanner Pizza decaf iced tea or coffee	1/2 ham & turkey sub on whole grain with Italian dressing & spicy mustard, 1 cup veggie soup decaf iced tea or coffee	pita fajita: chicken, peppers & onions decaf iced tea or coffee	pasta fagiole green salad with Italian dressing iced tea or coffee	turkey chili small spinach salad with rye crisp iced tea or coffee	veggie pocket sandwich with yogurt cheese iced tea or coffee	1/2 turkey club vegetable soup iced tea or coffee
PM snack	1 oz peanuts 1/2 cup apple juice	1 graham cracker with peanut butter 1/2 cup lowfat milk	1/2 celery stick with peanut butter 1/2 cup apple juice	lemonade sugar-free sweetener 1 slice yogurt cheese	1 oz peanuts 1 cup hot mulled cider	5-6 raw carrot sticks 1 oz peanuts	Hungarian cheese spread with saltine crackers
Dinner	salmon patties steamed broccoli macaroni & yogurt cheese decaf tea	barbecued chicken cole slaw Italian cut green beans decaf tea	oven fried catfish sauteed cabbage & onion, baked beets herb roll decaf tea	ham with mustard sauce steamed broccoli 1/2 baked yam decaf tea	broiled haddock with herbs steamed asparagus with low-fat hollandaise wild rice decaf tea	marinated flank steak red potato oven fries green salad decaf tea	sesame chicken 1/2 twice baked potato steamed spinach decaf tea
Dessert	mocha angel food cake decaf coffee	chocolate cake decaf coffee	carrot cake decaf coffee	1/2 cup low-fat banana pudding decaf coffee	low-fat chocolate mousse decaf coffee	small slice peanut butter pie decaf coffee	small slice cheese cake decaf coffee
Before-bed snack	cup of hot Ovaltine made with low fat milk	1/2 cup vanilla yogurt with a pinch of cinnamon	cup of hot Ovaltine made with low fat milk	1/2 cup apple juice 1 oz Swiss cheese	1 saltine cracker with peanut butter 1/2 cup cold low fat milk	cup of hot Ovaltine made with low fat milk	1/2 cup vanilla yogurt with a pinch of cinnamon

Remove this page and photocopy at 130% or contact Iron Disorders Institute for enlarged sheet

BLANK	MENU PLANNER						
	day one	day two	day three	day four	day five	day six	day seven
Breakfast							
AM snack							
Lunch							
PM snack optional							
Dinner							
Dessert							
Before-bed snack							

Remove this page and photocopy at 130% or contact Iron Disorders Institute for enlarged sheet

PHYTATE AND IRON-BINDING POLYPHENOLS *mg/100 g dry matter*

food item	phytate phosphorus	tannin equivalents	chlorogenic acid	TOTAL tannin equivalents
BEVERAGES:				
Coffee		21	71	55
Tea				
English Brkfst		53	14	60
Green		26	17	35
Herb		18		18
Cocoa				
Marabou	504	4400	520	4648
Dutch	513			
Swiss	481			
Beer				
Light lager		0.4		0.4
Whiskey				
Scotch		2.9		2.9
Wine				
White		0	4	2
Red		0.2 to 2.3	20-40	10-21
CEREALS, CRACKERS, BRAN, AND GRAINS:				
Cereals				
Corn flakes	12			
Millet	217			
Oats, rolled	282			
Semolina	19			
Sorghum				
Red	279	480		480
White	389	15		15
Wheat germ	467			
Flours				
Barley	185			
Oat	399-628			
Rice	27			
Wheat	680-1189		58	28
Crackers				
Rye, thin	72-86			
Rye fiber	114-193			
Graham	192			
Oat	166			
Rice cakes	113			

Beverage to Water Ratios:
coffee: 3.3 grams/100mL water or approx. 1oz/3.5 oz
tea: 1 gram /100mL water
Note: 1 milligram of phytate phosphorus= 3.5 milligrams phytic acid

Adopted from chart Hallberg and Hulthén (see bibliography)

PHYTATE AND IRON-BINDING POLYPHENOLS *mg/100 g dry matter*

food item	phytate phosphorus	tannin equivalents	chlorogenic acid	TOTAL tannin equivalents
CEREALS, CRACKERS, BRAN, AND GRAINS CONTINUED:				
Rice				
Long grain	53-64			
Wild, brown	181-215			
Spaghetti				
Barilla brand	71			
Buitoni brand	6			
FRUITS AND BERRIES:				
Apples	0.1	160		
Apricots				
Avocado	1.0			
Bananas	0.4	40		40
Blackberries	4.0	390		390
Blueberries	6.0	80		80
Currents				
Black	78.0			
Red	55.0			
Dates		5		5
Figs				5
Kiwi	10.0			
Cowberries	5.0	3	250	122
Mangos	1.0			
Melons, honey	0.6			
Oranges	2.0			
Pears	0.2	4	70	37
Raspberries	4.0	70	61	99
Rhubarb	0.2		16	8
Strawberries	4.0			

Note: 1 milligram of phytate phosphorus= 3.5 milligrams phytic acid

Adopted from chart Hallberg and Hulthén (see bibliography)

PHYTATE AND IRON-BINDING POLYPHENOLS *mg/100 g dry matter*

food item	phytate phosphorus	tannin equivalents	chlorogenic acid	TOTAL tannin equivalents
VEGETABLES:				
Asparagus				
Green	2			
White	3			
Beans				
Black	262			
Brown	195			
Green	15			
Mung	188	140		140
Red	271	1		1
White	269	0		0
Beets	2	3		3
Broccoli	10	1	40	20
Brussel sprouts	11			
Cabbage				
Chinese	2			
White	1			
Carrots	4		28	13
Cauliflower	3			
Celery	5			
Chicory	2			
Corn	24			
Cucumbers	1			
Eggplant	3	7	51	31
Garden cress	7			
Garlic	4		7	3
Horseradish	13			
Leeks	4		11	5
Lentils				
Brown	142	190		190
Red	122			
Lettuce,				
Iceberg	0.5			
Mushroom	13	1		1
Olives				
Black	3			
Onions				
Red	5	10		10
Yellow	16	6		6

Note: 1 milligram of phytate phosphorus= 3.5 milligrams phytic acid

Adopted from chart Hallberg and Hulthén (see bibliography)

PHYTATE AND IRON-BINDING POLYPHENOLS *mg/100 g dry matter*			
food item	phytate phosphorus	tannin equivalents	chlorogenic acid	TOTAL tannin equivalents

food item	phytate phosphorus	tannin equivalents	chlorogenic acid	TOTAL tannin equivalents
SPICES AND HERBS:				
Basil		2.7	7.9	6.5
Caraway		2.8	6.4	5.8
Cardamom		0.3		0.3
Cherval		0.4	2.0	1.4
Cinnamon		43.0	14.3	50.0
Clove		95.0		95.0
Cumin		2.8	6.4	5.8
Curry		6.2	9.9	10.9
Fennel		0.3		0.3
Ginger		0.2		0.2
Marjoram		6.4	9.9	11.1
Oregano	0.2	21.0	6.0	24.0
Pepper				
Black		2.0		2.0
Green		1.4		1.4
Red		0.4		0.8
White		0.4		0.4
Thyme		12.0	4.4	14.1
Turmeric		34.0	0.7	34.0
Vanilla		0.7		0.7
NUTS AND SEEDS:				
Almonds	296.0	43.0		43.0
Brazil nuts		10.0		10.0
Cashews				
Hazelnuts		256.0		256.0
Peanuts				
Walnuts	303.0	1400.0		1400.0
Linseeds	296.0	14.0		14.0
Sesame seeds	576.0			
Sunflower seeds	393	120		120

Note: 1 milligram of phytate phosphorus= 3.5 milligrams phytic acid

food item serving size	IRON* MILLIGRAMS		VITAMIN C MILLIGRAMS	FAT GRAMS	CARBOS GRAMS	FIBER GRAMS	PROTEIN GRAMS	CALORIES
	heme	nonheme						
BEVERAGES:								
Beer 8 oz	0.0	-	-	10.8	-	-	1.4	101
Whiskey								
(Scotch) 1 oz	0.0	0.0	-	-	t	-	-	70
Wine 4oz *								
Red dry	0.0	0.5	-	-	1 to 5	-	-	120
White dry	0.0	0.5	-	-	1 to 5	-	-	120
Sweet wines	0.0	0.5	-	-	8 to 9	-	-	120
Soft drinks 12 oz								
Lemon	0.0	0.2	-	-	36.2	-	-	144
Cola	0.0	0.1	-	-	40.0	-	-	154
Ginger ale	0.0	0.7	-	-	33.0	-	-	120
Root beer	0.0	0.2	-	-	42.0	-	-	154
Coffee (1 cup)	0.0	0.1	-	-	0.8	-	-	4
Tea (1 cup)	0.0	0.1	-	-	0.9	-	-	2

*Due to the great variety of wines these numbers represent typical amounts. Consult a more detailed food value composition reference list for specific wines.

CONDIMENTS/MISCELLANEOUS:								
Anchovy (3)	0.0	0.93	0.0	1.2	t	-	2.3	21
Bacon bits (¼ oz)	0.0	0.14	0.0	0.3	0.4	-	0.6	7
Barbecue sauce	0.14	0.7	0.3	5.0	-	-	0.2	15
Bouillon (1 cube)								
Beef	0.09	0.08	-	-	1.0	-	-	10
Chicken	0.09	0.08	-	-	1.0	-	-	10
Catsup	0.10	2.5	0.1	4.3	-	-	0.3	19
Garbanzo beans	1.60							
Horseradish			t	-	t	0.5	-	0.1 2
Mustard .	0.10	-	0.8	0.5	-	-	t	11
Olives (1 large)								
Black	0.09	-	0.8	1.0	-	-	-	10
Green	0.09	-	0.8	1.0	-	-	-	10
Pimento	0.00	0.20	t	0.6	0.1	-	0.1	3
Pickle (2 oz)								
Dill	0.0	0.35		t	0.3	0.1	t	1
Sweet	0.0	0.42		-	10.0	-	-	36
Soy sauce	0.0	0.49	-	-	0.9	-	-	10
Vinegar cider	0.0	0.10	-	-	1.0	-	-	2
Worcestershire	0.0	0.30	-	t	t	0.1	-	4

Serving sizes for condiments are one tablespoon unless otherwise specified.
*EXCEPT FOR KNOWN PERCENTAGES: Iron content values for meat are expressed as 40% heme and 60% nonheme.

food item* serving size	IRON MILLIGRAMS heme	nonheme	VITAMIN C MILLIGRAMS	FAT GRAMS	CARBOS GRAMS	FIBER GRAMS	PROTEIN GRAMS	CALORIES
BREADS:								
Biscuit	0.0	0.2	0.0	6.5	17.0		3.0	138
Cinnamon	0.0	0.7	0.0	3.0	15.0	2.0	2.0	90
Cornbread	0.0	1.2	0.0	7.0	29.0	1.7	4.0	200
English muffin	0.0	1.4	0.0	1.0	26.0	2.0	4.0	134
French bread	0.0	0.4	0.0	0.6	11.0		1.8	55
Pita pocket	0.0	1.4	0.0	2.0	33.0		6.0	165
Pumpernickel	0.0	0.8	0.0	4.0	17.0		2.9	79
Raisin	0.0	0.3	0.0	0.6	12.0		1.5	60
Rye	0.0	0.4	0.0	0.3	12.0		2.1	56
Taco shell	0.0	0.3	0.0	2.0	7.0	0.2	1.0	50
Tortilla,Corn	0.0	1.4	0.0	1.0	13.0	0.3	2.0	65
White	0.0	0.7	0.0	1.0	12.0	0.5	2.0	65
Whole wheat	0.0	1.0		1.0	13.0	1.4	3.0	70
CEREALS:								
Bran flakes	0.0	12.4	12.0	1.0	28.0	1.0	4.0	105
Corn flakes	0.0	1.8	15.0		24.0	0.4	2.0	110
Shredded Wheat		1.2		1.0	23.0	3.3	3.0	100
Rice (puffed)	0.0	0.3	0.0	0.1	12.5	0.2	1.0	54
Cream of wheat	0.0	8.2			22.0	0.6	3.0	105
Oatmeal	0.0	1.6		2.0	25.0	4.0	6.0	145
Cornmeal	0.0	4.2	0.0	2.0	43.0	6.8	4.0	210
Cornstarch 1tab	0.0	t		0.0	7.0		0.0	30
CRACKERS:								
Graham	0.0	0.4		1.0	11.0	2.8	1.0	60
Melba	0.0	0.1			4.0		1.0	20
Rye								
Saltine	0.0	0.5		1.0	9.0	0.5	1.0	50
FLOUR:								
Barley	0.0	6.6	0.0	4.0	135.0	32.0	23.0	651
Buckwheat	0.0	4.8	0.0	1.0	41.0	7.1	7.0	190
Oat	0.0	1.6	0.0	2.0	25.0	4.0	6.0	145
Rice	0.0	1.0	0.0	2.0	46.0	4.0	5.0	218
Rye	0.0	2.9	0.0	1.9	79.0		13.0	385
Wheat	0.0	4.6	0.0	2.2	87.1	15.1	16.4	407
Soy	0.0	5.7	0.0	2.4	33.4	3.7	40.9	287
PASTA AND SNACK FOODS								
Macaroni	0.0	2.1	0.0	1.0	39.0	1.2	7.0	190
Popcorn	0.0	0.3		3.0	6.0		1.0	55
Pretzels (per oz.)	0.0	0.3		1.0	13.0		2.0	65
RICE:								
Brown	0.0	0.5	0.0	1.0	25.0	2.4	2.0	115
White	0.0	0.9	0.0		25.0	0.1	2.0	110
Wild	0.0	1.0	0.0	0.6	35.0	0.5	6.5	166

Serving size for bread is one slice. All other portions are one cup unless otherwise specified.

*EXCEPT FOR KNOWN PERCENTAGES: Iron content values for meat are expressed as 40% heme and 60% nonheme.

food item serving size	IRON* MILLIGRAMS		VITAMIN C MILLIGRAMS	FAT GRAMS	CARBOS GRAMS	FIBER GRAMS	PROTEIN GRAMS	CALORIES
	heme	nonheme						
DAIRY:								
Cheese								
American	0.0	0.1	0.0	9.0	0.0	0.0	6.0	105
Bleu	0.0	0.2	0.0	9.0	1.0	0.0	6.0	103
Brie	0.0	0.1	0.0	7.0	0.0	0.0	6.0	85
Cheddar	0.0	0.2	0.0	9.0	0.0	0.0	7.0	113
Cottage								
1 cup	0.0	0.3	0.0	1.0	3.0	0.0	25.0	123
Cream								
1 tblsp.	0.0	0.2	0.0	5.0	0.0	0.0	1.0	51
Feta	0.0	0.1	0.0	6.0	1.1	0.0	4.0	75
Fontina	0.0	t	0.0	8.8	0.4	0.0	7.6	110
Gouda	0.0	t	0.0	7.8	0.6	0.0	8.5	101
Gruyere	0.0	0.3	0.0	8.9	0.5	0.0	8.1	115
Havarti								
Monterey								
jack	0.0	0.2	0.0	8.5	0.2	0.0	6.9	106
Mozzarella	0.0	t	0.0	4.5	0.7	0.0	6.9	72
Muenster	0.0	t	0.0			0.3	6.6	104
Neufchatel	0.0	t	0.0	6.6	0.8	0.0	2.8	74
Parmesan	0.0	0.1	0.0	7.3	0.8	0.0	10.0	110
Provolone	0.0	0.1	0.0	7.5	0.6	0.0	7.3	100
Ricotta (1 cup)	0.0	1.0	0.0	19.4	12.6	0.0	28.0	340
Swiss	0.0	0.2	0.0	7.9	0.5	0.0	7.8	99
Velveeta								
Cream (1 cup)								
Light	0.0	0.0	0.0	28.0	11.1	0.0	7.7	240
Heavy	0.0	0.0	0.0	90.0	7.4	0.0	5.2	861
Sour	0.0	0.0	0.0	43.2	8.0	0.0	6.4	456
Egg (1 lg)								
Yolk only	0.0	0.9	0.0	5.6	t	0.0	2.8	63
White only	0.0	0.1	0.0	0.0	0.4	0.0	3.3	16
Substitute								
1 oz	0.0	0.6	0.0	3.1	0.9	0.0	3.2	45
Ice cream (½ cup)								
plain	0.0	0.6	0.0	7.9	15.9	0.0	2.4	134
Ice milk	0.0	0.9	0.0	4.0	18.0	0.0	3.0	120
Frozen yogurt	0.0	0.1	0.0	1.0	23.0	0.0	3.0	120

Serving size is one ounce unless otherwise specified.

*EXCEPT FOR KNOWN PERCENTAGES: Iron content values for meat are expressed as 40% heme and 60% nonheme.

food item serving size	IRON* MILLIGRAMS		VITAMIN C MILLIGRAMS	FAT GRAMS	CARBOS GRAMS	FIBER GRAMS	PROTEIN GRAMS	CALORIES
	heme	nonheme						
DAIRY CONTINUED:								
Milk (1cup)								
Chocolate	0.0	0.6	0.0	8.5	25.9	0.2	7.9	208
Whole	0.0	0.1	0.0	8.2	11.4	0.0	8.0	150
2%	0.0	0.1	0.0	4.7	11.7	0.0	8.1	121
1%								
Skim	0.0	0.1	0.0	0.1	11.8	0.0	8.4	86
Buttermilk	0.0	0.1	0.0	2.2	11.7	0.0	8.1	99
Canned								
sweetened	0.0	0.5	0.0	26.6	166.5	0.0	24.2	982
condensed	0.0	0.6	0.0	19.1	25.3	0.0	17.2	338
Soy	0.0	1.3	0.0	4.6	4.3	2.6	7.0	79
Yogurt/low-fat								
Vanilla	0.0	t	t	2.8	31.3	0.0	11.2	194
FATS (ONE TABLESPOON):								
Butter		t	0.0	11.5			0.1	101
Margarine		0.0	0.0	11.4				101
Mayonnaise		0.1	0.0	11.0	0.4		0.2	99
Oils								
Canola			0.0	14.0				124
Corn			0.0	13.6				115
Olive			0.0	13.5				120
SALAD DRESSINGS:								
Bleu cheese			0.0	7.7	1.1		0.7	77
French		0.1	0.0	6.1	2.7	0.1	0.1	67
Italian			0.0	6.8	1.5		0.1	68
Ranch		0.1	0.0	5.0	1.0		0.0	50
Thousand Island		0.1	0.0	5.3	2.4	0.3	0.1	59

Serving size is one ounce unless otherwise specified.

*EXCEPT FOR KNOWN PERCENTAGES: Iron content values for meat are expressed as 40% heme and 60% nonheme.

food item serving size	IRON* MILLIGRAMS		VITAMIN C MILLIGRAMS	FAT GRAMS	per serving FOOD VALUES CARBOS GRAMS	FIBER GRAMS	PROTEIN GRAMS	CALORIES
	heme	nonheme						
FRUITS:								
Apples	0.0	0.25	8	0.5	21.0	1.0	0.2	81
Applesauce	0.0	0.29	2	0.1	27.5	1.3	0.4	106
Apricots	0.0							
Fresh	0.0	0.58	11	0.4	11.7	0.6	1.4	51
Dried (10 halves)	0.0	1.65	1	0.1	21.6	1.0	1.2	83
Avocados	0.0	2.05	24	30.8	14.8	4.2	4.0	324
Bananas	0.0	0.35	10	0.5	26.7	0.5	1.2	105
Blackberries	0.0	0.24	15	0.5	20.5	1.8	0.9	82
Blueberries	0.0	1.12	9	0.3	16.0	3.5	1.4	66
Cherries	0.0	0.56	5	1.4	24.0	0.6	1.7	104
Cranberries	0.0	0.19	13	0.2	12.0	1.1	0.3	46
Dates (10)	0.0	0.96	-	0.3	61.0	1.8	1.6	228
Grapefruit (½)	0.0	0.10	41	0.1	9.7	0.2	0.7	38
Grapes	0.0	0.30	5	0.3	15.7	0.7	0.5	58
Kiwi (1)	0.0	0.30	74	0.3	11.3	0.8	0.7	46
Limes (1 oz)	0.0	0.01	9	-	2.8	-	0.1	8
Mango	0.0	0.20	57	0.5	35.0	1.7	1.0	135
Melon (½)	0.0	0.50	58	0.7	22.0	0.9	2.3	94
Oranges	0.0	0.6	96	0.1	15.4	0.5	1.2	62
Peaches	0.0	0.1	12	-	9.6	0.5	0.6	37
Pears	0.0	0.2	7	0.6	25.0	2.3	0.6	98
Pineapples	0.0	0.6	24	0.6	19.2	0.8	0.6	77
Plums	0.0	0.1	12	0.4	8.6	0.4	0.5	36
Prunes (10)	0.0	2.0	4	-	52.7	1.7	2.1	201
Raisins	0.0	4.3	4	0.9	12.9	1.1	4.2	488
Raspberries	0.0	0.7	50	0.7	14.2	3.7	1.1	61
Strawberries	0.0	0.5	85	0.5	10.4	0.8	0.9	45
Watermelon	0.0	0.3	15	0.6	11.5	0.48	1.0	50

food item serving size	IRON* MILLIGRAMS		VITAMIN C MILLIGRAMS	FAT GRAMS	CARBOS GRAMS	FIBER GRAMS	PROTEIN GRAMS	CALORIES
	heme	nonheme						
BEEF:								
Brisket	0.55	1.6	0.0	14.2	0.1	0.0	21.8	222
Chuck roast	1.18	1.2	0.0	22.5	0.0	0.0	20.7	291
Dried beef (1oz)	0.64	0.6	0.0	1.1	4.4	0.0	8.2	47
Flank steak	0.55	1.6	0.0	14.2	0.1	0.0	21.8	222
Ground (lean)	0.8	1.2	0.0	9.7	0.0	0.0	5.0	224
Liver	3.0	4.6	0.0	4.3	6.5	0.0	22.6	161
Prime rib	0.95	0.9	0.0	33.0	0.0	0.0	18.2	375
Round steak	1.05	1.0	0.0	19.8	0.0	0.0	22.0	273
Sirloin	1.25	1.2	0.0	22.8	0.0	0.0	20.6	294
Tenderloin	1.35	1.3	0.0	20.4	0.0	0.0	21.0	275
POULTRY:								
Chicken (3.2 oz)								
Breast	0.4	0.7	0.0	4.2	0.0	0.0	27.0	154
Dark meat	0.5	0.8	0.0	10.0	0.0	0.0	27.0	203
Turkey								
Breast	0.4	0.7	0.0	3.5	0.0	0.0	29.8	91
Dark meat	0.5	0.8	0.0	4.0	0.0	0.0	16.0	104
PORK:								
Bacon (1 strip)	0.15	0.5	0.0	14.7	0.0	0.0	2.4	157
Canadian								
bacon	0.18	0.6	0.0	19.8	0.0	0.0	23.4	178
Ham	0.25	0.8	0.0	25.0	0.0	0.0	19.9	206
Pork chop (5oz)	0.18	0.6	0.0	43.0	0.0	0.0	20.0	345
Shoulder	0.25	0.8	0.0	25.7	0.0	0.0	18.2	312
Tenderloin	0.2	0.7	0.0	5.0	0.0	0.0	17.0	186
Roast	0.18	0.6	0.0	34.2	0.0	0.0	25.5	422
Spareribs	0.15	0.5	0.0	33.0	0.0	0.0	12.0	201
VENISON (3.2 oz.):	2.3	2.2	0.0	3.6	0.0	0.0	19.0	114
VEAL (3 oz):								
Breast	0.3	0.5	0.0	5.0	0.0	0.0	22.0	143
Roast	0.3	0.5	0.0	8.0	0.0	0.0	29.0	192

Serving size is 3 ounces unless otherwise specified.
*EXCEPT FOR KNOWN PERCENTAGES: Iron content values for meat are expressed as 40% heme and 60% nonheme.

food item serving size	IRON* MILLIGRAMS		VITAMIN C MILLIGRAMS	FAT GRAMS	CARBOS GRAMS	FIBER GRAMS	PROTEIN GRAMS	CALORIES
	heme	nonheme						
LUNCHEON MEAT:								
Beef bologna	0.1	0.2	-	9.1	0.4	0.5	3.3	89
Pork bologna	t	0.1	-	9.1	0.6	0.2	4.3	70
Italian sausage	0.4	0.6	-	8.9	0.2	0.0	4.0	98
Pepperoni	t	t	-	13.0	0.0	0.0	6.0	140
Polish sausage	0.1	0.2	-	8.1	0.5	0.0	4.0	92
Pork sausage	t	0.1	-	8.8	0.3	0.0	5.6	105
Pork salami	t	t	-	9.6	0.2	0.0	6.4	115
Turkey hot dog	t	0.1	-	5.0	0.4	0.0	4.1	64
MISCELLANEOUS:								

Serving size is one ounce unless otherwise specified.
*EXCEPT FOR KNOWN PERCENTAGES: Iron content values for meat are expressed as 40% heme and 60% nonheme.

food item serving size	IRON* MILLIGRAMS		VITAMIN C MILLIGRAMS	*per serving* FOOD VALUES				
	heme	nonheme		FAT GRAMS	CARBOS GRAMS	FIBER GRAMS	PROTEIN GRAMS	CALORIES
NUTS AND SEEDS:								
Almonds	0.0	6.7	0.0	77	27.7	3.8	26.4	849
Cashews	0.0	5.3	0.0	64	41.0	1.9	24.1	785
Coconut	0.0	1.4	0.0	28.2	7.5	2.7	2.8	277
Hazelnuts	0.0	4.6	0.0	84.2	22.5	1.1	17.0	856
Macadamia nuts	0.0	3.2	0.0	98.8	18.4	7.1	11.0	940
Peanuts	0.0	3.2	0.0	70.1	29.7	3.9	37.7	838
Pecans	0.0	2.6	0.0	76.9	15.8	2.3	9.9	742
Pistachios	0.0	8.6	0.0	61.9	31.7	2.4	26.0	739
Pumpkin seeds	0.0	15.7	0.0	65.4	21.0	2.7	40.6	774
Sesame seeds	0.0	3.6	0.0	80	26.4	3.6	27.3	873
Sunflower seeds	0.0	10.3	0.0	68.6	28.9	5.5	34.8	812
Walnuts	0.0	3.1	0.0	64	15.8	2.1	14.8	651
Peanut butter	0.0	0.3	0.0	8.1	3.2	0.3	3.9	86
MISCELLANEOUS:								

Serving size is one ounce unless otherwise specified.
*EXCEPT FOR KNOWN PERCENTAGES: Iron content values for meat are expressed as 40% heme and 60% nonheme.

food item serving size	IRON*		VITAMIN C	FAT	FOOD VALUES CARBOS	FIBER	PROTEIN	CALORIES
	MILLIGRAMS		MILLIGRAMS	GRAMS	GRAMS	GRAMS	GRAMS	
	heme	nonheme						
SEAFOOD:								
Anchovies (5)	0.37	0.5	0	1.9	0.0	0	5.8	42
Catfish	0.4	0.6	0	3.6	0.0	0	15.5	99
Caviar (1T)	0.7	1.0	0	2.8	0.6	0	3.9	40
Clams (9)	10.0	15.0	0	0.6	4.6	0	23.0	130
Cod	t	0.1	0	0.6	0.0	0	15.0	70
Crab	0.2	0.3	0	0.5	0.0	0	15.6	71
Haddock	0.4	0.6	0	0.6	0.0	0	16.0	70
Halibut	0.3	0.4	0	2.0	0.0	0	17.7	93
Herring	0.4	0.5	0	7.7	0.0	0	15.0	134
Lobster	0.2	0.3	0	0.7	0.4	0	16.0	77
Mackerel	0.5	0.8	0	2.8	0.0	0	22.8	114
Oysters (6)	2.2	3.3	0	2.1	0.0	0	5.9	58
Perch	0.3	0.5	0	1.4	0.0	0	15.8	80
Pollack	0.2	0.2	0	0.8	0.0	0	16.4	75
Salmon	0.3	0.4	0	6.0	0.0	0	17.0	121
Sardines (2)	0.3	0.4	0	2.7	0.0	0	5.9	50
Scallops	t	0.1	0	0.6	0.0	0	14.3	75
Shrimp	0.8	1.2	0	1.5	0.0	0	17.3	90
Snails (escargot)	1.7	2.6	0	0.3	0.0	0	6.6	20
Snapper	t	t	0	1.0	0.0	0	17.4	85
Swordfish	0.3	0.4	0	3.4	0.0	0	16.8	103
Trout	0.5	0.8	0	5.6	0.0	0	17.7	126
Tuna	1.1	1.7	0	0.6	0.0	0	20.0	94
Whitefish	0.1	0.1	0	5.0	0.0	0	16.0	114

Serving size is 3 ounces unless otherwise specified.
*EXCEPT FOR KNOWN PERCENTAGES: Iron content values for meat are expressed as 40% heme and 60% nonheme.

food item serving size	IRON* MILLIGRAMS		VITAMIN C MILLIGRAMS	FAT GRAMS	CARBOS GRAMS	FIBER GRAMS	PROTEIN GRAMS	CALORIES
	heme	nonheme						
VEGETABLES:								
Artichoke	0.0	1.1	8.0	0.2	9.9	6.0	2.8	44
Asparagus								
(1 spear)	0.0	0.1	5.3	0.6	0.6	-	0.3	16
Beans								
Black	0.0	5.2	0.0	1.0	40.8	7.2	15.2	226
Green	0.0	0.7	0.2	8.9	10.0	4.0	2.0	44
Kidney	0.0	5.2	2.0	1.0	40.0	13.0	15.0	225
Lima	0.0	4.4	0.0	1.0	42.0	14.0	15.0	229
Navy	0.0	2.5	0.0	0.0	19.0	4.0	7.0	109
Pinto	0.0	2.2	2.0	0.4	43.6	6.8	14.0	234
Beets	0.0	0.5	5.0	t	5.7	0.7	0.9	26
Broccoli	0.0	0.6	58.0	0.2	3.9	2.0	2.3	22
Brussels								
sprouts	0.0	0.5	0.5	0.4	6.8	3.4	2.0	30
Cabbage	0.0	0.2	18.0	0.1	1.9	0.4	0.4	8
Carrots	0.0	0.2	2.0	0.1	5.6	1.8	0.6	24
Cauliflower	0.0	0.2	36.0	0.1	2.9	1.4	1.2	15
Celery	0.0	0.2	4.0	0.1	2.2	1.0	0.5	10
Collards	0.0	0.1	8.0	t	1.3	0.1	0.3	6
Corn	0.0	0.5	5.0	1.1	20.6	3.0	2.7	89
Cucumber	0.0	0.1	2.0	0.1	1.5	0.5	0.3	7
Eggplant	0.0	0.2	1.0	0.1	3.2	0.5	0.4	13
Garlic (1 clove)	0.0	t	1.0	t	1.0	0.1	0.2	4
Kale	0.0	0.6	27.0	0.3	3.7	0.5	1.2	21
Kohlrabi	0.0	0.3	44.0	0.1	5.5	0.9	1.5	24
Leeks	0.0	0.6	2.0	0.2	7.4	0.6	0.8	32
Lettuce								
Bibb	0.0	0.5	13.0	0.1	0.7	0.3	0.4	4
Iceberg	0.0	0.3	1.0	0.1	0.6	0.3	0.3	4
Leaf	0.0	0.4	5.0	0.1	1.0	0.2	0.4	5
Romaine	0.0	0.3	7.0	0.1	0.7	0.5	0.5	4
Mushrooms	0.0	0.4	1.0	0.2	1.6	0.5	0.7	9
Mustard greens	0.0	0.5	10.0	0.1	1.4	0.2	0.8	7
Okra	0.0	0.4	13.0	0.1	3.8	0.5	1.0	25
Onions	0.0	0.2	5.0	0.1	6.9	1.3	0.9	30
Parsley	0.0	1.8	27.0	0.1	2.1	1.3	0.7	10
Parsnips	0.0	0.4	10.0	0.2	15.2	2.1	1.0	63
Peas	0.0	1.2	11.0	0.2	12.5	3.0	4.3	67
Peppers								
Green	0.0	0.2	45.0	0.1	3.2	0.8	0.4	13
Red	0.0	0.2	95.0	0.1	3.2	0.8	0.4	13

Serving size is one half cup unless otherwise specified.
*EXCEPT FOR KNOWN PERCENTAGES: Iron content values for meat are expressed as 40% heme and 60% nonheme.

food item _serving size_	IRON* _MILLIGRAMS_		VITAMIN C _MILLIGRAMS_	FAT _GRAMS_	CARBOS _GRAMS_	FIBER _GRAMS_	PROTEIN _GRAMS_	CALORIES
	heme	nonheme						
VEGETABLES CONTINUED:								
Peppers								
Green	0.0	0.2	45.0	0.1	3.2	0.8	0.4	13
Red	0.0	0.2	95.0	0.1	3.2	0.8	0.4	13
Potatoes								
Sweet	0.0	0.7	25.0	0.1	24.3	3.0	1.7	103
White	0.0	0.8	26.0	0.1	24.4	1.0	2.2	105
w/skin	0.0	2.7	15.0	0.2	51.0	5.3	4.7	220
Pumpkin	0.0	0.7	6.0	0.1	6.0	1.0	0.9	24
Radishes (10)	0.0	0.1	10.0	0.2	1.6	0.2	0.3	7
Sauerkraut	0.0	1.7	17.0	0.2	5.1	1.3	1.0	22
Spinach	0.0	0.7	8.0	0.1	1.0	0.7	0.8	6
Squash	0.0	0.6	8.0	t	8.0	3.0	1.0	29
Tomatoes	0.0	0.4	17.0	0.3	4.2	1.2	0.8	19
Zucchini	0.0	0.3	4.0	0.1	1.9	0.3	0.8	9
MISCELLANEOUS:								

Serving size is one cup unless otherwise specified.
*EXCEPT FOR KNOWN PERCENTAGES: Iron content values for meat are expressed as 40% heme and 60% nonheme.

Food Diary		DAY:			WEEK:		

Food item portion size	IRON heme non-heme milligrams		vitaman C milligrams	FAT grams	CARBS grams	PROTEIN grams	CALORIES
TOTALS							

Iron Disorders Institute Iron Diary Form 2008

SHOPPING LIST

*USE A HIGHLIGHTER TO NOTE
WHICH FOODS YOU WISH TO PURCHASE*

Produce:
Lettuce
Romaine
Iceberg
Bibb
Other:
Cabbage
Green
Savoy
Red
Onion
Yellow
White
Vidalia
Spring
Spinach
Chives
Parsley
Tomatoes
Cucumbers
Radishes
Asparagus
Beans
Cauliflower
Broccoli
Squash
Peas
Potatoes
Red
Sweet
Idaho/russet

Fruit:
Apples
Grapes
Cherries
Peaches
Pears
Strawberries
Blueberries
Raspberries
Blackberries
Pineapple
Oranges
Watermelon
Melon
Kiwi
Banana

Dairy:
Sour cream
Milk
Buttermilk
Heavy cream
Light cream
Butter
Yogurt
Eggs

Cheeses:
Monterey jack
Mozzarella
Parmesan
Swiss
Fontina
Havarti
Cheddar
Other:

Meat:
Chicken breast
Chicken dark meat
Chicken whole
Turkey breast
Turkey breast-ground
Turkey dark meat
Turkey whole
Veal cutlets
Veal ground
Veal roast
Veal stew meat
Ham steak
Ham picnic shoulder
Pork filet
Pork roast
Pork stew meat
Pork ground
Beef-sirloin ground
Beef sirloin steak
Beef filet

Fish:
Bass
Flounder
Grouper
Halibut
Mackerel
Perch
Orange roughy
Salmon
Shrimp
Snapper
Sole
Swordfish
Tuna
Trout

Frozen:
Yogurt
Pie crust
Vegetables:

Dry goods:
Flour
Cornmeal
Beans
Rice
Pasta

Spices/herbs:
Bay leaf
Basil
Cumin
Greek
Garlic
Marjoram
Oregano
Rosemary
Red pepper
black pepper
White pepper
Sage
Salt
Thyme
Cinnamon
Nutmeg
Ginger

Canned goods:
Tomates diced
Tomato paste
Tomato sauce

Oils/Condiments:
Apple cider vinegar
Brown sugar
Catsup
Coffee
Olive oil
Olives
Tea

Other:
_____
_____
_____
_____
_____
_____
_____
_____
_____
_____
_____
_____
_____
_____
_____
_____
_____
_____
_____

The Recipes

Important: The sample menu planners and recipes in The Hemochromatosis Cookbook *are suggestions. Menu planning and changes in diet should be discussed with a healthcare provider and nutritionist, especially for hemochromatosis diabetes patients. Patients with liver disease should limit excessive consumption of tannins, which can be harmful to a liver that is damaged or compromised.*

Clam Spread

2 tablespoons canned minced clams, drained and rinsed
1 tablespoon apple juice
4 ounces Neufchâtel cheese
¼ cup diced Velveeta cheese
1 tablespoon finely chopped onion
1 tablespoon finely chopped green pepper
1 teaspoon Worcestershire sauce
   Pinch red pepper

In a food processor combine all of the ingredients. Pulse until well blended.

Spread on melba toast rounds and place under the broiler to heat.

Serves 4

THIS RECIPE

is LOW in HEME iron and contains the following substances that inhibit absorption of nonheme iron:

✓ calcium
✓ dairy phosphate
eggs
✓ phytate phosphorus
POLYPHENOLS
tannic acid
chlorogenic acid
✓ phenolic acid
oxalates

PER SERVING

IRON	heme iron	nonheme iron
	0.2 mg	0.4 mg

"Crab" Spread

1   cup chopped imitation crab
1   tablespoon apple juice
1   spring onion, chopped
1   8-ounce package Neufchâtel
     cheese
     Pinch red pepper
2   tablespoons chopped fresh
     parsley
1   tablespoon finely chopped onion

In a large bowl combine all of the ingredients with hands. Refrigerate until chilled.

Serve chilled on saltine crackers.

Serves 4

THIS RECIPE

is LOW in HEME iron and contains the following substances that inhibit absorption of nonheme iron:

✓ calcium

✓ dairy phosphate

eggs

✓ phytate phosphorus

POLYPHENOLS

✓ tannic acid

✓ chlorogenic acid

phenolic acid

oxalates

PER SERVING

IRON	heme iron	nonheme iron
	0.0 mg	0.5 mg

Hungarian Cheese Spread

¼ cup (½ stick) butter, softened
1 package cream cheese, softened
1 tablespoon caraway seed
1 tablespoon ground paprika
1 tablespoon chives
1 teaspoon dry mustard
2 tablespoons finely chopped green pepper
¼ cup chopped radishes

In a medium bowl combine all of the ingredients. Serve chilled on saltine crackers or rye or wheat bread.

Serves 4

THIS RECIPE

is LOW in HEME iron and contains the following substances that inhibit absorption of nonheme iron:

✓ calcium
✓ dairy phosphate
eggs
✓ phytate phosphorus
POLYPHENOLS
tannic acid
chlorogenic acid
phenolic acid
✓ oxalates

PER SERVING

IRON	heme iron	nonheme iron
	0.0 mg	trace

Refried Beans

1 pound pinto beans
2 quarts water
1 tablespoon instant coffee
2 ounces country ham
2 tablespoons olive oil
   Pinch red pepper

THIS RECIPE

is LOW in HEME iron and contains the following substances that inhibit absorption of nonheme iron:

calcium

✓ dairy phosphate

eggs

✓ phytate phosphorus

POLYPHENOLS

✓ tannic acid

✓ chlorogenic acid

phenolic acid

oxalates

PER SERVING

IRON	heme iron	nonheme iron
	trace	4.5 mg

Rinse and clean the beans thoroughly. Bring the beans to a boil in the water. Add the coffee and ham, boil for 10 minutes, then reduce the heat to simmer. Cover and slow cook for 2 hours.

Check each 40 minutes or so to assure adequate liquid still remains.

Remove the ham and cool the beans. Taste the beans for saltiness. (*Note:* Country ham is very salty; if another type of ham is used salt may need to be added for seasoning.)

In a food processor purée the beans. Drizzle the oil into the mixture. Add the red pepper. Add remaining liquid as needed to keep a paste-like texture.

Makes 6 1-cup servings

Avocado Dip

¼ cup chopped onion
2 avocado, peeled and seed
  removed
2 tablespoons apple juice (to retard
  oxidation of avocado)
½ cup diced fresh tomato
½ cup sour cream
1 teaspoon salt
  Pinch red pepper

In a food processor pulse the onion until finely chopped. Add the avocado and apple juice, and mix. Add the tomato, sour cream, salt, and pepper. Pulse until all is blended well.

**Yield 2½ cups;
serving size: ¼ cup**

THIS RECIPE

*is LOW in HEME iron and contains
the following substances that
inhibit absorption of nonheme iron:*

✓ calcium

✓ dairy phosphate

eggs

✓ phytate phosphorus

POLYPHENOLS

tannic acid

chlorogenic acid

✓ phenolic acid

oxalates

PER SERVING

IRON	heme iron	nonheme iron
	0.0 mg	0.9 mg

Banana-Pineapple Cooler

1   medium banana, not overripe
¼   cup fresh pineapple
½   cup apple juice
1   teaspoon sugar
½   cup pineapple sherbet

In a blender combine all ingredients and blend on high speed.

Serve over ice.

Serves 1

THIS RECIPE

is LOW in HEME iron and contains the following substances that inhibit absorption of nonheme iron:

calcium

dairy phosphate

eggs

phytate phosphorus

POLYPHENOLS

✓ tannic acid

✓ chlorogenic acid

✓ phenolic acid

oxalates

PER SERVING

IRON	heme iron	nonheme iron
	0.0 mg	0.6 mg

Faux Whiskey Sour

½ cup brewed tea
2 ounces Wild Turkey whiskey
2 tablespoons frozen lemonade

THIS RECIPE

is LOW in HEME iron and contains the following substances that inhibit absorption of nonheme iron:

	calcium
	dairy phosphate
	eggs
	phytate phosphorus

POLYPHENOLS

✓ tannic acid
✓ chlorogenic acid

	phenolic acid
	oxalates

PER SERVING

IRON	heme iron	nonheme iron
	0.0 mg	0.1 mg

In a small saucepan combine all of the ingredients and bring to a boil. Remove from the heat and place in the freezer to cool.

Serve over cracked ice.

Note: Alcohol enhances the absorption of iron, and frequent consumption of alcoholic beverages can cause liver disease. Alcohol has a lower boiling point than water and so by bringing the liquid to a boil the alcohol content is burned out without losing the flavor of the whiskey.

Serves 1

Fresh-Squeezed Lemonade

¾   cup sugar

¾   cup hot water

1   cup lemon juice (about 12 lemons)

7   cups water

In a pitcher dissolve the sugar in the hot water. Add the lemon juice and water. Stir and serve over ice.

Serves 8

THIS RECIPE

is LOW in HEME iron and contains the following substances that inhibit absorption of nonheme iron:

calcium

dairy phosphate

eggs

phytate phosphorus

POLYPHENOLS

✓ tannic acid

✓ chlorogenic acid

phenolic acid

oxalates

PER SERVING

IRON	heme iron	nonheme iron
	0.0 mg	0.1 mg

Hot Cocoa

6   tablespoons cocoa powder
6   tablespoons sugar
    Dash salt
1   cup water
2   cups milk
1   cup light cream or half and half

THIS RECIPE

*is LOW in HEME iron and contains
the following substances that
inhibit absorption of nonheme iron:*

✓ calcium

✓ dairy phosphate

eggs

phytate phosphorus

POLYPHENOLS

✓ tannic acid

✓ chlorogenic acid

phenolic acid

oxalates

PER SERVING

IRON	heme iron	nonheme iron
	0.0 mg	trace

In a saucepan combine the cocoa, sugar, salt, and water. Bring to a boil, stirring constantly with a wooden spoon until liquid will coat the back of the spoon. Reduce the heat and stir in the milk. Add the cream. Serve with marshmallows or whipped cream topping.

Chocolate contains high levels of tannins and chlorogenic acid; this old-fashioned recipe is a good alternative to a cup of coffee or tea.

Serves 6

Mulled Cider

2 quarts apple cider
½ cup brown sugar
1¼ teaspoons ground cinnamon
1¼ teaspoons allspice
1 tablespoon whole cloves

In a saucepan simmer the cider on the stovetop. Add the sugar and spices, and bring to a gentle boil. Cover, cut off the heat, and steep for 20 minutes. Do not remove the cover until 20 minutes have lapsed.

Serves 8

THIS RECIPE

is LOW in HEME iron and contains the following substances that inhibit absorption of nonheme iron:

calcium

dairy phosphate

eggs

phytate phosphorus

POLYPHENOLS

✓ tannic acid

✓ chlorogenic acid

✓ phenolic acid

oxalates

PER SERVING

IRON	heme iron	nonheme iron
	0.0 mg	0.6 mg

Peach Frost

½ **cup sliced fresh peaches**
½ **cup apple juice**
1 **cup frozen vanilla yogurt**

In a blender combine all of the ingredients and blend well. Serve in a tall chilled glass.

Serves 1

This Recipe

is LOW in HEME iron and contains the following substances that inhibit absorption of nonheme iron:

calcium

✓ dairy phosphate

eggs

phytate phosphorus

POLYPHENOLS

✓ tannic acid

✓ chlorogenic acid

phenolic acid

oxalates

Per Serving

IRON	heme iron	nonheme iron
	0.0 mg	0.1 mg

Raspberry Faux Champagne

2   cups chilled white grape juice

2   cups chilled ginger ale

4   tablespoons frozen raspberries with syrup

In a pitcher mix all of the ingredients together. Serve in fluted glasses.

Serves 4

THIS RECIPE

is LOW in HEME iron and contains the following substances that inhibit absorption of nonheme iron:

calcium

dairy phosphate

eggs

phytate phosphorus

POLYPHENOLS

✓ tannic acid

✓ chlorogenic acid

✓ phenolic acid

oxalates

PER SERVING

IRON	heme iron	nonheme iron
	0.0 mg	0.3 mg

Spiced Chocolate Shake

1½ cups milk
2 tablespoons instant coffee
½ teaspoon ground cinnamon
¼ teaspoon ground cloves
2 cups chocolate ice cream
Chocolate shavings

In a blender combine all ingredients. Blend until combined. Serve in chilled glasses with chocolate shavings as garnish.

Serves 4

THIS RECIPE

is LOW in HEME iron and contains the following substances that inhibit absorption of nonheme iron:

✓ calcium

✓ dairy phosphate

eggs

phytate phosphorus

POLYPHENOLS

✓ tannic acid

✓ chlorogenic acid

✓ phenolic acid

oxalates

PER SERVING

IRON	heme iron	nonheme iron
	0.0 mg	0.4 mg

Coffee

Coffee was first cultivated in Arabia more than five hundred years ago. During the sixteenth and seventeenth centuries, coffee from the islands of Mocha and Java was introduced all over Europe, where coffeehouses became commonplace. American coffeehouses were first established as early as 1689 in Boston, New York, and Philadelphia.

Most coffees are derived from two species of beans: arabica and robusta. Arabicas offer the finest aroma and flavor, are less acidic, and have less caffeine than robustas coffees. American coffees are of the robusta beans. Coffees are labeled by either the darkness of the roast or by the region where the bean was grown. The majority of coffee is grown in Africa, Central and South America, and Indonesia. It is also grown in Hawaii, the Caribbean, New Guinea, India, and the Middle East.

Coffee beans are picked green and roasted, which provides the rich flavor.

Roasting typically takes from 1 to 17 minutes at temperatures between 380° and 480°F. The longer the roast, the deeper the flavor and color of the beans. The degree of roast is designated by names such as American and French Roast. Roast time and temperature also depend on moisture content and density of the beans.

Tannin or tannic acid contained in coffee can inhibit the absorption of nutrients, especially minerals such as iron. Tannin makes up about 8 percent of a green coffee bean and is what gives coffee its bite.

Coffee can also stimulate the production of stomach acid, which probably accounts for the reason why tea is a better inhibitor of iron absorption than coffee. Studies demonstrate that one cup of strong coffee drank within two hours of meal consumption impaired absorption of iron up to 60 percent, while tea can inhibit iron absorption by as much as 80 to 90 percent.

How to Brew Coffee

There are three basic brewing methods: drip, vacuum, and percolator, but all methods require 1 tablespoon of coffee to 8 ounces of water, unless stronger coffee is preferred.

Drip coffee method: Water is poured into a reservoir where it is heated and flows over coffee contained in a basket. Brewed coffee drips into a glass pot.

Vacuum coffee method: Hot water is placed in the upper portion of a two-part glass or metal coffee maker. The hot water is pressed over the coffee and forced into the bottom portion of the maker.

Percolator method: Coffeemakers are usually electric. Water is placed in the coffee-maker and a basket containing coffee is held by a stem that is inserted into the pot. The boiling water percolates up through the stem, pouring onto the coffee and seeping out into the water below.

Espresso is a method of brewing more than a type of coffee. Although one can purchase coffee labeled espresso, the term comes from the Italian word meaning "fast."

Espresso was invented in 1903 by Luigi Bezzera, the owner of a manufacturing business. He was not happy because his employees were taking too long for their coffee breaks. In an effort to shorten breaks and increase productivity Bezzera found a way to shorten the brewing process used to make traditional coffee. He invented a machine that used pressure in the brewing process, reducing the time needed to brew a pot of coffee. He called his new machine the "Fast Coffee Machine," which would make a cup of coffee in just 20 seconds.

Café Vienna

4 cups strong hot coffee plus 1 tablespoon instant coffee

½ cup heavy cream

¼ cup Faux Molasses, or to taste (see page 258)

½ teaspoon ground cinnamon

Pour the coffee into a clean tea pot or coffee carafe. Dissolve the instant coffee in the hot coffee.

Add cream, syrup, and cinnamon.

Garnish each serving with a dollop of whipped cream and a sprinkle of cinnamon, and serve promptly.

Serves 4

THIS RECIPE

is LOW in HEME iron and contains the following substances that inhibit absorption of nonheme iron:

✓ calcium

✓ dairy phosphate

eggs

✓ phytate phosphorus

POLYPHENOLS

✓ tannic acid

✓ chlorogenic acid

phenolic acid

oxalates

PER SERVING

IRON	heme iron	nonheme iron
	0.0 mg	0.7 mg

The Hemochromatosis Cookbook

Iced Coffee

4 cups brewed coffee

2 tablespoons instant coffee

3 tablespoons Faux Molasses (see recipe on page 258)

½ cup milk

In a pitcher combine the coffee, molasses, and milk. Pour over ice. Serve with a straw.

Serves 4

THIS RECIPE

is LOW in HEME iron and contains the following substances that inhibit absorption of nonheme iron:

✓ calcium

✓ dairy phosphate

eggs

✓ phytate phosphorus

POLYPHENOLS

✓ tannic acid

✓ chlorogenic acid

phenolic acid

oxalates

PER SERVING

IRON	heme iron	nonheme iron
	0.0 mg	0.6 mg

Mocha Café Latte

2   cups strong coffee
2   cups scalded milk
4   tablespoons Nestle's brand instant cocoa

In a saucepan combine the coffee, milk, and cocoa. Mix well. Serve in warm mugs.

Serves 4

Iced Mocha Café Latte

2   cups strong coffee
2   tablespoons instant coffee
2   cups scalded milk
6   tablespoons Nestle's brand instant cocoa

In a saucepan combine the brewed coffee, instant coffee, milk, and cocoa. Cool and serve over ice.

Serves 4

THESE RECIPES

are LOW in HEME iron and contain the following substances that inhibit absorption of nonheme iron:

✓ calcium
✓ dairy phosphate
eggs
✓ phytate phosphorus
POLYPHENOLS
✓ tannic acid
✓ chlorogenic acid
phenolic acid
oxalates

PER SERVING

IRON	heme iron	nonheme iron
	0.0 mg	0.7 mg

Tea

According to Chinese legend, tea has been around for more than five thousand years. During this ancient period, the emperor ruled that all drinking water was to be boiled as a hygienic precaution. One summer day while traveling, servants to the emperor were preparing a pot of boiling water. Dried tea leaves accidentally landed in the pot. Curious about the taste, the emperor drank the concoction and reported that he felt good afterward. And so, according to legend, tea was created.

From China, tea was introduced to Japan by a returning Buddhist priest and to Europe by a Portuguese Jesuit missionary. Tea was transported by the Portuguese to Lisbon and Dutch ships transported it to France, Holland, and the Baltic countries.

In the 1600s tea became popular throughout Europe, Russia, and the American colonies. Russian interest in tea began as early as 1618. Dutch explorer Peter Stuyvesant brought the first tea to America in 1650 to the colonists in the Dutch settlement of New Amsterdam (later renamed New York by the English). The first samples of tea reached England between 1652 and 1654. Tea quickly proved popular enough to replace ale as the national drink of England.

Today American schoolchildren learn about the famous Boston Tea Party where our colonial forefathers protested the British tea tax, an act that eventually led to the start of the Revolutionary War. During this century, two major American contributions to the tea industry occurred. In 1904, iced tea was created at the World's Fair in St. Louis, and in 1908, Thomas Sullivan of New York developed the concept of tea in a bag.

All tea comes from an evergreen shrub called the Camellia sinensis plant. Even though there are more than 1,500 different blends of tea, all blends are derived from just three types of tea: black, green and oolong. The difference comes in how the tea leaves are processed. Tea leaves are picked and rolled then allowed to wither and then to ferment or oxidize. The dark substances that form while the tea leaves are exposed to the air are produced by the chemical reactions of the tannins in the tea. They give the tea astringency, robust flavor, and aroma, and they leach into hot water to produce the characteristic reddish amber color. The oxidizing stage of tea processing does not take long, no more than four hours. When the leaves have transformed sufficiently, then they are "fired," dried over heat to stop the oxidation process. The length of time leaves oxidize determines the type of tea.

Black tea ferments the longest; well-known types of black tea include: orange pekoe, Darjeeling, Earl Grey, and English breakfast.

Green tea skips the oxidizing step. Instead, the leaves are steamed right after the withering stage, which destroys the enzymes that would otherwise cause the darkening. The steamed leaves are rolled and immediately fired.

Because the tannins do not go through the oxidizing process, which has a mellowing effect, green tea can be bitter and more astringent than black, especially if it is steeped for a long time.

Oolongs are "semi-fermented" teas. That is, they are processed the same way black teas are, but they aren't allowed to oxidize fully.

Herbal teas are not true teas. They are infusions or tisane (tee-zonh), which is French for "herbal drink." Popular infusions include rose hips, peppermint, and chamomile. Some herbal "teas" provide health benefits and some, such as peppermint, contain substances (possibly oxalates) that inhibit the absorption of nonheme iron.

Health Benefits of Drinking Tea
Scientists continue to report findings that iron excesses can contribute to heart disease and nourish cancer cells and that drinking tea reduces the risk of these chronic illnesses. Teas contain tannins and chlorogenic acid, two polyphenols that inhibit the absorption of nonheme iron. Polyphenols are powerful antioxidants, which combat free radical activity.

How to Brew Tea
In a saucepan bring fresh cold water to a full rolling boil. Measure 1 teaspoon of tea or 1 tea bag per cup of water. Cut off the heat and drop the tea bags into the water. Allow tea to steep 3 to 5 minutes, depending on the strength you like.

Note: If using loose tea, cheesecloth or a tea infuser can hold the tea while it steeps, or hot water can be poured directly over the tea leaves and strained after steeping. Remove the tea bags and add sugar if desired. Do not add sugar to boiling water, this can cause an injury.

Cranberry Cherry Tea

8 cups brewed tea
½ cup grenadine
1 cup cranberry juice

In a pitcher combine all of the ingredients. Serve over ice.

Serves 8 to 10

THIS RECIPE

is LOW in HEME iron and contains the following substances that inhibit absorption of nonheme iron:

calcium

dairy phosphate

eggs

phytate phosphorus

POLYPHENOLS

✓ tannic acid

✓ chlorogenic acid

phenolic acid

✓ oxalates

PER SERVING

IRON	heme iron	nonheme iron
	0.0 mg	0.6 mg

Lemon Tea

¾   cup sugar
¾   cup hot water
1   cup lemon juice (about 12 lemons)
7   cups brewed tea

THIS RECIPE

is LOW in HEME iron and contains the following substances that inhibit absorption of nonheme iron:

calcium

dairy phosphate

eggs

phytate phosphorus

POLYPHENOLS

✓ tannic acid

✓ chlorogenic acid

phenolic acid

oxalates

PER SERVING

IRON	heme iron	nonheme iron
	0.0 mg	0.4 mg

In a saucepan dissolve the sugar in the hot water. Set aside.

In a separate pan boil water to brew the tea. As the water boils, add the lemon juice. Allow the lemon water to boil rapidly for 20 to 30 seconds before adding the tea bags. Cut off the heat; allow the tea to steep. When fully steeped, stir in the sugar water and serve over ice.

Serves 8 to 10

Lime Zinger

2   **tablespoons sugar**
7   **cups brewed green tea**
¾   **cup lime juice**
3   **cups ginger ale**

In a pitcher dissolve the sugar in the warm tea. Add the lime juice and ginger ale.

Serve over ice.

Serves 8

This Recipe

is LOW in HEME iron and contains the following substances that inhibit absorption of nonheme iron:

calcium

dairy phosphate

eggs

phytate phosphorus

POLYPHENOLS

✓ tannic acid

✓ chlorogenic acid

phenolic acid

oxalates

Per Serving

IRON	heme iron	nonheme iron
	0.0 mg	0.7 mg

Spiced Tea (Hot or Iced)

4   cups water
1   family-sized Lipton brand tea bag
½   teaspoon each: cinnamon, cloves, ginger
4   tablespoons sugar
2   cups apple cider
      Cinnamon sticks

THIS RECIPE

is LOW in HEME iron and contains the following substances that inhibit absorption of nonheme iron:

calcium

dairy phosphate

eggs

phytate phosphorus

POLYPHENOLS

✓ tannic acid

✓ chlorogenic acid

✓ phenolic acid

oxalates

PER SERVING

IRON	heme iron	nonheme iron
	0.0 mg	0.4 mg

In a saucepan bring the water to a boil. Pour over the tea bag and spices, and steep for 4 to 5 minutes. Add the sugar, and stir to dissolve. Add the cold apple cider. Serve over ice.

To serve hot: Heat the apple cider in the microwave or on the stovetop and add to steeped tea and spice mixture. Serve in warm mugs with cinnamon sticks.

Serves 8

Soups & Stews

Stocks or Broths

Important bases for soups and sauces

Vegetable broth: When preparing vegetables such as onions, celery (including celery leaves), carrots, tomatoes, kelp, spinach, kale, etc. (wash greens thoroughly), toss ends or leftovers in stockpot filled with 14 to 16 cups of water. Add 4 to 6 crushed garlic cloves (okay to include skins), 1 teaspoon each: basil, rosemary, thyme, oregano, and salt, and 1/4 teaspoon white pepper. Simmer until all vegetables are tender (about 45 minutes to 1 hour); let stand to cool. Strain the vegetables and place the broth in a glass container.

Meat stock: Bones and organ meats are rich in hemoglobin/heme iron. Prepare stock using the fatty parts of the meats rather than carcass or bony parts such as neck and back, or organ meats. Strain the broth and refrigerate so the fat congeals on top and can be removed before use in soups and sauces.

Simmer fatty boneless meat scraps in 12 to 14 cups water. Season with 1 teaspoon of salt, 1 medium whole onion, and 2 tablespoons chopped fresh parsley. Simmer uncovered for 2½ hours. Cool, remove the meat, strain the broth, and refrigerate. Discard the meat.

Chicken or turkey stock: Simmer fatty boneless white and dark chicken or turkey meat in 12 to 14 cups of water. Season with 1 teaspoon of salt, 1 medium whole onion, and 2 tablespoons chopped fresh parsley. Simmer uncovered for 2½ hours. Cool, remove and reserve the meat for soups, salads, or casseroles. Before use in soups or sauces, strain the broth and refrigerate so the fat congeals on top and can be removed before use in soups and sauces.

Seafood stock: Simmer 1 pound of favorite fish (fillet) and 1 cup cleaned and deveined raw small shrimp in 12 to 14 cups water. Season with 1 teaspoon of salt, 1 medium whole onion, celery with leaves, and 2 tablespoons chopped fresh parsley. Simmer uncovered for 2½ hours. Cool, remove the meat, strain the broth, and refrigerate. Cool the strained fish, shrimp, and seasonings, and reserve for seafood lasagna.

Cream of Broccoli Soup

1   bunch fresh broccoli with stems (about 5 cups)
4   cups turkey or chicken broth
1   cup brewed tea
     Salt to taste
4   ounces Neufchâtel cheese (cream cheese)
1½   cups lowfat milk
½   cup olive oil
2   tablespoons butter
½   cup flour
1   cup light cream
¼   teaspoon nutmeg
⅛   teaspoon red pepper

THIS RECIPE

is LOW in HEME iron and contains the following substances that inhibit absorption of nonheme iron:

	✓ calcium
	✓ dairy phosphate
	eggs
	✓ phytate phosphorus
	POLYPHENOLS
	✓ tannic acid
	✓ chlorogenic acid
	phenolic acid
	✓ oxalates

PER SERVING

IRON	heme iron	nonheme iron
	0.0 mg	1.1 mg

Rinse the broccoli well. Cut and set aside about ⅔ cup of florets (tiny). Coarsely chop the stems (except for very ends) and remaining florets.

In a saucepan simmer the broccoli in the broth along with the tea and salt to taste until tender, about 15 to 20 minutes.

Cool well, then purée in a blender about 2 cups at a time (if not properly cooled the mixture can spew out when the blender is in operation). Return the puréed broccoli and broth to the warm saucepan. Add the diced Neufchâtel cheese and blend. Add the milk and bring the mixture to a gentle boil over medium-high heat.

In a medium saucepan heat the oil and butter. Whisk in the flour until a paste is formed. Slowly pour the broccoli and broth mixture into the paste, whisking until smooth. Add the cream, nutmeg, and pepper. Add the florets and simmer until the florets are tender. Do not boil once the cream is added.

Serves 8

Cream of Celery and Fennel Soup

½ cup olive oil
1 cup finely chopped onions
1 cup chopped celery, including tops
1 cup chopped fennel, including tops
2 tablespoons butter
½ cup flour
5 cups turkey or chicken broth
1 cup brewed tea
½ cup finely chopped fresh spinach
4 ounces Neufchâtel cheese, diced
1½ cups milk
1 cup light cream
1 teaspoon salt
⅛ teaspoon white pepper

In a medium saucepan heat the oil and sauté the onions. Add the celery and fennel and sauté until tender.

In a separate pan heat the butter. Whisk in the flour until a paste is formed. Slowly add the broth to the paste, mixing well. Add the tea. Transfer the sautéed onion, celery, and fennel to the soup mixture. Add the spinach and Neufchâtel cheese, and blend well. Add the milk and bring the mixture to a gentle boil over medium-high heat. Add the cream, salt, and pepper and heat through. Do not boil once the cream is added.

Serves 8

This Recipe

is LOW in HEME iron and contains the following substances that inhibit absorption of nonheme iron:

✓ calcium
✓ dairy phosphate
eggs
✓ phytate phosphorus
POLYPHENOLS
✓ tannic acid
✓ chlorogenic acid
phenolic acid
✓ oxalates

Per Serving

IRON	heme iron	nonheme iron
	trace	0.4 mg

Cream of Chicken Soup

½ cup olive oil
2 tablespoons butter
½ cup flour
6 cups turkey or chicken broth
1 tablespoon instant tea
1 cup pulled chicken meat
4 ounces Neufchâtel cheese, diced
1½ cups lowfat milk
1 cup light cream
¼ teaspoon nutmeg
⅛ teaspoon red pepper

In a medium saucepan heat the oil and butter, and whisk in the flour until a paste is formed. Slowly add the broth to paste, mixing well. Add the tea, chicken, and diced Neufchâtel cheese, and blend well. Add the milk and bring the mixture to a gentle boil over medium-high heat. Add the cream, nutmeg, and pepper, and heat through. Do not boil once the cream is added.

Serves 8

THIS RECIPE

is LOW in HEME iron and contains the following substances that inhibit absorption of nonheme iron:

✓ calcium

✓ dairy phosphate

eggs

✓ phytate phosphorus

POLYPHENOLS

✓ tannic acid

✓ chlorogenic acid

phenolic acid

✓ oxalates

PER SERVING

IRON	heme iron	nonheme iron
	0.4 mg	1.1 mg

Pepper Soup

2 tablespoons olive oil

1 small onion, chopped (⅓ cup)

¼ cup flour

4 cups vegetable or chicken broth

1 cup brewed tea

1 small green pepper, chopped (½ cup)

1 small red sweet pepper, chopped (½ cup)

4 ounces Neufchâtel cheese, diced

1 cup milk

½ cup light cream

1 teaspoon chives

¼ teaspoon salt

¼ teaspoon black pepper

¼ teaspoon ground red pepper

In a stockpot heat the oil and sauté the onion until tender, about 20 minutes. Whisk in the flour until a paste is formed. Slowly add the broth to the paste. Add the tea, peppers, and diced Neufchâtel cheese and blend. Add the milk and heat to a gentle boil. Reduce the heat and add the cream, chives, salt, and black and red peppers. Do not boil once the cream is added.

Serves 6

THIS RECIPE

is LOW in HEME iron and contains the following substances that inhibit absorption of nonheme iron:

✓ calcium

✓ dairy phosphate

eggs

✓ phytate phosphorus

POLYPHENOLS

✓ tannic acid

✓ chlorogenic acid

phenolic acid

oxalates

PER SERVING

IRON	heme iron	nonheme iron
	0.0 mg	0.4 mg

Potato and Leek Soup

6	cups russet potatoes
2	tablespoons olive oil
2	chopped leeks
1	cup finely chopped celery
7	cups vegetable stock or water
1	cup brewed tea
2	teaspoons salt
4	tablespoons dried instant mashed potatoes
1	cup milk
1	cup light cream
2	tablespoons chives
1	teaspoon black pepper

Wash the potatoes; peel and cut in large chunks. Reserve in cold water.

In a stockpot heat the oil and sauté the leeks until tender. Add the celery and cook until tender. Add the stock (or water), tea, salt, and russet potatoes, and simmer for about 40 minutes or until the potatoes are done.

Add the instant potatoes and milk and simmer until the soup is hot. Add the cream, chives, and pepper.

Serves 8

THIS RECIPE

is LOW in HEME iron and contains the following substances that inhibit absorption of nonheme iron:

✓ calcium

✓ dairy phosphate

eggs

✓ phytate phosphorus

POLYPHENOLS

✓ tannic acid

✓ chlorogenic acid

phenolic acid

oxalates

PER SERVING

IRON	heme iron	nonheme iron
	0.0 mg	0.77 mg

The Hemochromatosis Cookbook

Red Potato and Pepper Soup

2   tablespoons olive oil
1/2   cup chopped onion
1/2   cup diced green pepper
1/4   cup pimientos, drained
1   cup brewed tea
3   cups broth
1   teaspoon salt
1/4   teaspoon black pepper
12   red potatoes, washed and quartered
2   cups lowfat milk
1/4   to 1/2 cup instant mashed potatoes
1/2   cup sour cream
1   tablespoon chopped chives

In a stockpot heat the oil and sauté the onion until tender, about 15 minutes.

Add the green pepper, and simmer for 5 to 6 minutes. Stir in the pimientos and heat through. Add the tea, broth, salt, pepper, and potatoes. Simmer until the potatoes are tender.

Add the milk and instant potatoes until the desired thickness. Stir in the sour cream and chives.

Serves 8

THIS RECIPE

is LOW in HEME iron and contains the following substances that inhibit absorption of nonheme iron:

✓ calcium

✓ dairy phosphate

eggs

✓ phytate phosphorus

POLYPHENOLS

✓ tannic acid

✓ chlorogenic acid

phenolic acid

oxalates

PER SERVING

IRON	heme iron	nonheme iron
	0.0 mg	0.35 mg

Turkey Rice Soup

2	tablespoons olive oil
1/2	cup chopped onion
1/2	cup chopped celery
1	cup brewed tea
7	cups turkey broth
1/4	cup chopped fresh spinach
1/8	cup shredded carrots
1/2	cup uncooked basmati rice
1	tablespoon chives
1	tablespoon salt
1/8	teaspoon black pepper
1 1/2	cups chopped turkey meat

In a stockpot heat the oil and sauté the onion until tender. Add the celery and cook for 5 minutes. Add the tea, broth, spinach, carrots, rice, chives, salt, pepper, and meat. Simmer until the rice is tender.

Serves 8

THIS RECIPE

is LOW in HEME iron and contains the following substances that inhibit absorption of nonheme iron:

calcium

dairy phosphate

eggs

phytate phosphorus

POLYPHENOLS

✓ tannic acid

chlorogenic acid

phenolic acid

✓ oxalates

PER SERVING

IRON	heme iron	nonheme iron
	0.44 mg	2.37 mg

Vegetable Soup

2 tablespoons olive oil
½ cup finely chopped onion
1 cup chopped green cabbage
½ cup coarsely chopped celery, including leaves
1 cup diced tomatoes
5 cups water
1 cup hot tea
½ can tomato paste (3 ounces)
1 teaspoon basil
2 teaspoons salt
1 teaspoon black pepper
¼ cup corn
¼ cup green peas
½ cup green beans
½ cup parsnips
½ cup diced potatoes

In a stockpot heat the oil and sauté the onion until tender. Add the cabbage and celery and cook until the cabbage is wilted. Add the diced tomatoes and bring to a boil for 10 minutes until the tomatoes are tender. Add the water, tea, tomato paste, seasonings, and all vegetables. Simmer partially covered for 1½ hours.

Serves 6

THIS RECIPE

is LOW in HEME iron and contains the following substances that inhibit absorption of nonheme iron:

✓ calcium
✓ dairy phosphate
✓ eggs
✓ phytate phosphorus

POLYPHENOLS
✓ tannic acid
✓ chlorogenic acid
✓ phenolic acid
✓ oxalates

PER SERVING

IRON	heme iron	nonheme iron
	trace	0.8 mg

Vegetable Soup with Meat

¼ cup olive oil
½ cup finely chopped onions
¾ pound trimmed veal stew meat
   Flour to coat meat
¼ cup olive oil
1 teaspoon salt
1 teaspoon black pepper
2 cups Progresso brand crushed tomatoes with sauce
2 quarts water
1 tablespoon instant coffee
1 medium potato, peeled and cubed
1 cup sliced okra
½ cup lima beans
1 cup corn

In a stockpot heat ¼ cup of olive oil and sauté the onions for about 20 minutes.

Cut the meat into large cubes. Dredge the meat in flour. Add the remaining oil to the onions, heat, and brown the meat in the hot oil. Season the cooked meat with salt and pepper. Add the tomatoes, water, coffee, and vegetables, and simmer for 1½ hours.

Serves 8

THIS RECIPE

is LOW in HEME iron and contains the following substances that inhibit absorption of nonheme iron:

calcium

dairy phosphate

eggs

phytate phosphorus

POLYPHENOLS

✓ tannic acid

chlorogenic acid

phenolic acid

oxalates

PER SERVING

IRON	heme iron	nonheme iron
	0.3 mg	0.7 mg

Seafood Chowder

1   quart water
1   tablespoon instant tea
¼   pound shelled and deveined shrimp
2   tablespoons olive oil
½   cup finely chopped onion
1   28-ounce can diced tomatoes
3   cups broth
2   tablespoons chopped fresh chives
2   bay leaves
¼   teaspoon thyme
1   tablespoon salt
1   teaspoon coarse black pepper
4   red-skinned potatoes, scrubbed and quartered
½   cup instant potatoes
½   pound haddock fillets cut into large pieces
1   pint light cream

In a stockpot boil 1 quart of water plus 1 tablespoon of instant tea. Drop in the shrimp, and cook about 5 minutes. The shrimp will curl when done; if over-cooked, shrimp are tough.

Remove the shrimp, set aside, and reserve the broth.

In a skillet heat the olive oil and sauté the onion for about 15 minutes. Add the tomatoes and simmer another 15 minutes.

Add the broth, seasonings, and potatoes, and simmer 30 minutes.

Add the instant potatoes, then the haddock, and simmer 20 minutes.

Add the cream and cooked shrimp, and heat but do not boil.

Serves 6

THIS RECIPE

is LOW in HEME iron and contains the following substances that inhibit absorption of nonheme iron:

✓ calcium

✓ dairy phosphate

eggs

✓ phytate phosphorus

POLYPHENOLS

✓ tannic acid

✓ chlorogenic acid

phenolic acid

oxalates

PER SERVING

IRON	heme iron	nonheme iron
	0.6 mg	2.1 mg

Hot Beef Stew

1   pound of lean sirloin beef
1   cup of brewed green tea
¼   cup flour
¼   cup olive oil
1   cup chopped onion
1   can beef broth
1   cup burgundy red wine
8   red potatoes cut in halves
4   carrots, washed and cut into large pieces
1   teaspoon salt
5–6   shakes of red pepper flakes (or to taste)

Cut beef into large chunks and marinate overnight in green tea.

Remove beef from marinade (do not discard) and place in a zip-top plastic bag; add flour and shake until meat is coated.

In a large pot heat the olive oil and sauté the onion until golden brown, then add the meat. Cook until meat is done, about 20 minutes.

Slowly add reserved marinade, beef broth, and then wine.

Bring to boil. Add potatoes, carrots, salt, and red pepper flakes. Reduce heat and simmer for 1 hour.

Serves 4 to 6

THIS RECIPE

is HIGH in HEME iron and contains the following substances that inhibit absorption of nonheme iron:

calcium

dairy phosphate

eggs

phytate phosphorus

POLYPHENOLS

✓ tannic acid

chlorogenic acid

phenolic acid

oxalates

PER SERVING

IRON	heme iron	nonheme iron
	1.1 mg	1.2 mg

Chicken Salad

3   chicken breasts plus 1 thigh/leg piece, cooked and cooled
2   quarts water
1   tablespoon instant tea
3   hard boiled eggs
¼   cup green pepper
¼   cup celery
3   tablespoons Hellman's brand re-duced-fat mayonnaise
1   teaspoon yellow mustard
¼   teaspoon salt
⅓   cup sweet pickle relish

THIS RECIPE

is LOW in HEME iron and contains the following substances that inhibit absorption of nonheme iron:

calcium
✓ dairy phosphate
eggs
✓ phytate phosphorus
POLYPHENOLS
✓ tannic acid
✓ chlorogenic acid
phenolic acid
oxalates

PER SERVING

IRON	heme iron	nonheme iron
	0.4 mg	0.8 mg

In a stockpot simmer the chicken in the water with the instant tea for 1 hour.

Remove the chicken and place in the refrigerator to cool. Reserve the broth for other recipes.

When the chicken is completely cooled (40° to 45°F. center temperature), pull from the bone, taking care to remove all cartilage, fat, and skin. Watch for small bones. Place the chicken in a food processor and chop until coarse. Place the chopped chicken in a large mixing bowl. Chop the boiled eggs in the food processor, pulsing until coarse; add to the mixing bowl. Chop the green pepper and celery in the food processor, pulsing until coarse; add to the mixing bowl (peppers and celery will clean the egg from the bowl of processor). Add the mayo 1 tablespoon at a time, and add the yellow mustard, salt, and sweet pickle relish. Mix thoroughly. Add tiny amounts of mayo until the desired consistency is reached. Refrigerate before serving.

Serve as a cold plate with pasta salad and cottage cheese.

Serves 4 to 6

Diet Turkey Salad

2 cups cold, cooked white turkey meat
¼ green pepper, cut into pieces
1 stalk celery, cut into pieces
2 tablespoons chopped onion
3 cooked egg whites
3 tablespoons Hellman's brand reduced-fat mayonnaise
Dash salt (optional)

In a food processor pulse the turkey meat until chopped. Remove and set aside.

In the food processor place the green pepper, celery, and onion, and pulse until coarsely ground. Add to the turkey. In the processor chop the egg whites. Transfer to the turkey mixture. Add the mayonnaise and mix thoroughly. Season with salt to taste.

Serves 4 to 6

THIS RECIPE

is LOW in HEME iron and contains the following substances that inhibit absorption of nonheme iron:

calcium
✓ dairy phosphate
✓ eggs
✓ phytate phosphorus
POLYPHENOLS
✓ tannic acid
✓ chlorogenic acid
phenolic acid
oxalates

PER SERVING

IRON	heme iron	nonheme iron
	0.1 mg	0.2 mg

Broccoli Cauliflower Salad

1   cup fresh broccoli florets
1   cup cauliflower florets
1   cup mayonnaise
1   tablespoon sugar
2   tablespoons apple cider vinegar
¼   cup crumbled crisp bacon
½   cup celery

In a salad dish combine the broccoli and cauliflower. In a small bowl combine the mayonnaise, sugar, and vinegar with a whisk. Pour over the broccoli and cauliflower and stir in the bacon and celery.

Serves 4 to 6

THIS RECIPE

is LOW in HEME iron and contains the following substances that inhibit absorption of nonheme iron:

✓ calcium

✓ dairy phosphate

eggs

✓ phytate phosphorus

POLYPHENOLS

tannic acid

chlorogenic acid

phenolic acid

✓ oxalates

PER SERVING

IRON	heme iron	nonheme iron
	0.0 mg	0.4 mg

Cole Slaw

½   **head cabbage**
¼   **green pepper**
1   **rib celery**
¼   **cup sliced onion**
¼   **cup sliced carrot**
½   **cup mayonnaise**
¼   **cup cider vinegar**
¼   **teaspoon salt**
¼   **cup sugar**

Wash the cabbage, cut into pieces, and place in a food processor. Pulse until finely chopped, and transfer to a large bowl. Place the green pepper, celery, onion, and carrot in the processor, and pulse until coarse. Add to the chopped cabbage.

In a separate bowl whisk together the mayonnaise, vinegar, salt, and sugar. Pour into the cabbage mixture and blend. Refrigerate until ready to serve.

Serves 4

THIS RECIPE

is LOW in HEME iron and contains the following substances that inhibit absorption of nonheme iron:

✓ calcium
✓ dairy phosphate
eggs
✓ phytate phosphorus
POLYPHENOLS
tannic acid
chlorogenic acid
phenolic acid
oxalates

PER SERVING

IRON	heme iron	nonheme iron
	trace	0.5 mg

Layered Salad

½ cup mayonnaise

1 cup sour cream

3 cups chopped lettuce (romaine and iceberg work best)

⅔ cup chopped raw cauliflower

⅔ cup chopped raw broccoli

½ cup frozen small peas

½ cup coarsely chopped walnuts

4 spring onions, washed, trimmed, and diced (reserve tops)

½ cup finely chopped celery

2 cups shredded sharp Cheddar cheese

6 strips crisp bacon or Webb's "Faux Bacon" (see page 201)
Salt to taste

In a small bowl mix the mayonnaise and sour cream to create a sauce.

In a glass dish alternate layers of lettuce, cauliflower, broccoli, peas, walnuts, onions, celery, sauce, cheese, and bacon, ending with cheese and bacon as the final layers. Sprinkle salt as desired onto the lettuce layers. Refrigerate until serving.

Serves 6

THIS RECIPE

is LOW in HEME iron and contains the following substances that inhibit absorption of nonheme iron:

✓ calcium

✓ dairy phosphate

eggs

✓ phytate phosphorus

POLYPHENOLS

✓ tannic acid

✓ chlorogenic acid

phenolic acid

✓ oxalates

PER SERVING

IRON	heme iron	nonheme iron
	trace	1.26 mg

Macaroni Salad

½ cup mayonnaise
2 tablespoons sugar
3 tablespoons cider vinegar
½ teaspoon salt
2 quarts water
½ teaspoon salt
1 tablespoon instant tea
2 cups dry elbow macaroni
¼ cup finely chopped onion
½ cup finely chopped celery
2 boiled eggs, chopped

In a small bowl whisk together the mayonnaise, sugar, vinegar, and ½ teaspoon of salt.

In a stockpot bring the water to a boil. Add ½ teaspoon of salt, the tea, and macaroni, and cook for 10 minutes. Drain and rinse.

While the noodles are still warm add the mayonnaise mixture, onion, celery, and eggs. Cover and refrigerate for several hours; overnight is best.

Serves 8

THIS RECIPE

is LOW in HEME iron and contains the following substances that inhibit absorption of nonheme iron:

calcium
✓ dairy phosphate
✓ eggs
✓ phytate phosphorus
POLYPHENOLS
✓ tannic acid
chlorogenic acid
phenolic acid
oxalates

PER SERVING

IRON	heme iron	nonheme iron
	trace	0.67 mg

Pasta Salad

DRESSING:

2 tablespoons olive oil
1 tablespoon cider vinegar
1 teaspoon salt
1 teaspoon garlic powder
¼ teaspoon oregano
¼ teaspoon basil

SALAD:

1 16-ounce box whole-wheat rotini pasta
2 quarts water
1 tablespoon instant tea
1 teaspoon salt
2 pickling cucumbers, cubed
1 cup tomato relish
6 ounces Provolone cheese, cut into small cubes
⅔ cup sliced black olives
4 ounces hard salami, cut into thin strips
½ cup Parmesan cheese

In a shaker combine the olive oil, cider vinegar, and remaining ingredients. Shake until well combined.

In a large pot cook the pasta in the water and tea with salt until tender.

Drain, rinse, and toss with dressing. Add the cucumbers and tomato relish, and toss. Add the Provolone, olives, salami, and Parmesan. Chill before serving.

Serves 10 to 12

THIS RECIPE

is LOW in HEME iron and contains the following substances that inhibit absorption of nonheme iron:

✓ calcium

✓ dairy phosphate

eggs

✓ phytate phosphorus

POLYPHENOLS

✓ tannic acid

✓ chlorogenic acid

phenolic acid

oxalates

PER SERVING

IRON	heme iron	nonheme iron
	0.5 mg	0.56 mg

Potato Salad

3	pounds red skinned potatoes
2	quarts water
1	teaspoon salt
1	tablespoon instant tea
½	cup mayonnaise
1	tablespoon yellow mustard
¼	cup sugar
¼	cup apple cider vinegar
¼	cup finely chopped onion
½	cup finely chopped celery
2	chopped hard-boiled eggs

Rinse the potatoes. In a stockpot boil the potatoes in salted water with the tea for about 40 minutes.

In a small bowl combine the mayonnaise, mustard, sugar, and vinegar.

Drain and cut each potato in half. Place in a salad bowl. While still warm, add the onion, celery, eggs, and mayonnaise mixture. Combine thoroughly and refrigerate before serving.

Serves 10 to 12

THIS RECIPE

is LOW in HEME iron and contains the following substances that inhibit absorption of nonheme iron:

calcium

✓ dairy phosphate

eggs

✓ phytate phosphorus

POLYPHENOLS

✓ tannic acid

✓ chlorogenic acid

phenolic acid

oxalates

PER SERVING

IRON	heme iron	nonheme iron
	0.0 mg	0.5 mg

Tuna Salad

3   pounds red skinned potatoes
2   quarts water
1   teaspoon salt
1   tablespoon instant tea
½   cup mayonnaise
1   tablespoon yellow mustard
¼   cup sugar
¼   cup apple cider vinegar
¼   cup finely chopped onion
½   cup finely chopped celery
2   chopped hard-boiled eggs

Rinse the potatoes. In a stockpot boil the potatoes in salted water with the tea for about 40 minutes.

In a small bowl combine the mayonnaise, mustard, sugar, and vinegar.

Drain and cut each potato in half. Place in a salad bowl. While still warm, add the onion, celery, eggs, and mayonnaise mixture. Combine thoroughly and refrigerate before serving.

Serves 10 to 12

PER SERVING

IRON	heme iron	nonheme iron
	0.21 mg	0.7 mg

Honey Mustard

1   cup mayonnaise
¼   cup spicy mustard
¼   cup honey

PER SERVING

IRON	heme iron	nonheme iron
	trace	0.1 mg

In a small bowl combine all of the ingredients and mix well with a whisk.

Honey mustard can be used as a spread for sandwiches, a dipping sauce for vegetables or meat, or a salad dressing. reduced-fat mayonnaise can be substituted.

Serving size: 2 tablespoons

Italian Dressing

2   tablespoons olive oil
1   tablespoon cider vinegar
¾   teaspoon salt
½   teaspoon garlic powder

PER SERVING

IRON	heme iron	nonheme iron
	0.0 mg	0.09 mg

In a shaker with a tight-fitting lid combine all of the ingredients. Shake until blended.

Pour onto salad for four and toss well until all lettuce is coated. The secret is in the tossing.

Serves 4

Low-Calorie Herb and Cucumber Dressing

1   small pickling cucumber, washed and cut in chunks
½   cup Hellman's brand lowfat mayo
¼   cup cider vinegar
¾   teaspoon salt
½   teaspoon garlic powder
1   teaspoon chives
½   teaspoon parsley
¼   teaspoon marjoram
¼   teaspoon oregano

In a food processor pulse the cucumber until finely chopped. Add the mayonnaise and mix well. Add the cider vinegar and remaining ingredients, and blend well.

**Makes about ¾ cup;
serves 6**

THIS RECIPE

*is LOW in HEME iron and contains
the following substances that
inhibit absorption of nonheme iron:*

calcium

dairy phosphate

eggs

phytate phosphorus

POLYPHENOLS

tannic acid

chlorogenic acid

phenolic acid

✓ oxalates

PER SERVING

IRON	heme iron	nonheme iron
	trace	0.01 mg

Oil-Free Salad Dressing

½   cup cold brewed tea
1   teaspoon Knox unflavored gelatin
1   cup boiling water
¼   cup red wine vinegar
1   tablespoon spicy mustard
½   teaspoon paprika
1   teaspoon garlic powder
1   teaspoon dried parsley flakes
1   teaspoon salt
¼   teaspoon black pepper

In a blender combine the cold tea and gelatin. Add the boiling water and process at low speed until the gelatin is completely dissolved. Add the remaining ingredients and continue blending on low speed until combined. Place in a glass jar with a lid and refrigerate.

Shake well before serving.

**Makes about 2 cups;
serving size 2 tablespoons**

THIS RECIPE

*is LOW in HEME iron and contains
the following substances that
inhibit absorption of nonheme iron:*

calcium

dairy phosphate

eggs

phytate phosphorus

POLYPHENOLS

✓ tannic acid

chlorogenic acid

phenolic acid

✓ oxalates

PER SERVING

IRON	heme iron	nonheme iron
	trace	0.8 mg

Breads

Legend is that the sandwich was invented in the mid 1700s by an English nobleman whose title was the Earl of Sandwich, so derived from the name of the town Sandwich. It seems the Earl requested that a slab of meat be served between two slices of bread, which was a novel approach to eating one's dinner. His motive seemed to be driven by his love of playing cards. Eating in this way he could have one hand free so that he could hold his cards in the other. Another legend is that an English housewife weary of the consequences of greasy fingers and the constant cleaning associated with mealtime, slathered a creamy concoction we know today as mayonnaise onto two slices of bread, which also held a slab of meat.

In any event, bread is a necessary component of the traditional American sandwich, which today can be made in a variety of ways. Pockets, wraps, shells, and interesting breads such as Ezekiel and other multigrain breads add fiber to the diet and uniqueness of taste and texture.

Bread dates back to ancient Egypt, where more than four thousand years ago bakers discovered the qualities of yeast; until then bread was unleavened. Bread was often made in the home using wholegrain flours, although bakeries were commonplace throughout Europe and the USA. During Civil War times there were more than 2,000 bakeries in America. It was also during this time that the invention of specialized milling equipment allowed commercial bakeries to refine flour and produce lighter breads. After World War II few homemakers made bread at home; instead they purchased commercially produced breads that by now lined the shelves of grocery stores. For aesthetics commercial bakeries refined the grains, milling away the bran portion of the wheat. They spun air into the dough to give it a light and delicate texture and they added preservatives to extend the shelf life of the product. In the 1940s bakers began to add fortificants such as iron to commercially made bread. Americans consumed this type of bread for decades until the benefits of consuming whole grains led to the restoration of whole-grain breads in great variety. However, fortificants such as iron continue to be added to most commercially produced breads.

All breads contain nonheme iron, some more than others, especially those heavily fortified with iron. Whole-grain breads are high in insoluble fiber (part of phytates), which causes this iron to have low bioavailability. However, two fortificants that will soon make their way into our food supply, Ferrochel and EDTA-Fe, have the ability to override the iron-inhibitory capabilities of fiber. Individuals with iron-loading conditions will need to pay special attention to foods fortified with these substances. Meanwhile, enjoy sandwiches made with breads such as bagels, whole grains, and pita pockets, and try to drink tea or coffee with sandwiches.

Bagel: a roll made of yeast dough that is rolled and twisted into a doughnut shape, dropped into boil water to swell, and then is baked.

Biscuit: made of lard or vegetable shortening such as Crisco, which is cut into flour, to which buttermilk is added.

English muffin: rolled dough cut into circles and sprinkled with cornmeal are cooked on a very hot iron skillet, which accounts for its higher than baked bread iron content.

Ezekiel bread: called the Bible bread, it is an ancient bread that is low in gluten. It is made with sprouted grains, which include wheat, smelt, millet, barley, lentil, and soy flour. This bread also contains soya lecithin, which is thought to aid in the control of low-density cholesterol.

French or Italian bread: crusty bread with soft, airy center

Kaiser roll: same texture as French or Italian bread except in a roll form and usually topped with poppy seed. Also referred to as hard roll.

Millet bread: a good alternative grain for those who are allergic to wheat. It contains no gluten.

Pita pocket: an ancient flatbread common in the Mediterranean.

Pumpernickel: a coarse, dark bread made with unsifted rye, also called Westphalian rye, popular in Germany.

Rye: having its distinct flavor derived from caraway seed, rye bread is another German bread.

Taco shell: made from corn.

Tortilla: flat unleavened corn cake common in Mexico.

White: usually made from refined white flours, which does not contain the bran portion of the grain.

Whole wheat: contains the bran portion of the grain.

Some sandwiches in the *Hemochromatosis Cookbook* are from the roster of favorites served in my restaurant. To add novelty to the menu, most of the sandwiches were given silly names based on the names of famous people. This list includes José Felisalami, Veggie Jackson, Nickolettuce and Aleggsandria, Ike 'n' Tina Tuna, and Frankenstein's Muenster. Some sandwiches were named after favorite songs such as "Don't Go Bacon My Heart," "Fool's Russian In, " and "Pig O My Heart."

Applesauce Zucchini Bread

1   cup coarsely grated apples
2   tablespoons apple juice
1½ cups oat blend flour
¼   teaspoon salt
1   teaspoon baking soda
1   cup light brown sugar
1   cup apple butter
1   egg, lightly beaten
½   cup buttermilk
½   cup chopped zucchini
½   cup chopped English walnuts

THIS RECIPE

is LOW in HEME iron and contains the following substances that inhibit absorption of nonheme iron:

✓ calcium

✓ dairy phosphate

✓ eggs

✓ phytate phosphorus

POLYPHENOLS

✓ tannic acid

✓ chlorogenic acid

✓ phenolic acid

oxalates

PER SERVING

IRON	heme iron	nonheme iron
	0.0 mg	0.4 mg

In a small bowl sprinkle the apples with apple juice. Set aside.

In a medium bowl sift together the flour, salt, and baking soda.

In a large bowl blend the sugar, apple butter, and egg. Alternate adding dry ingredients and buttermilk to the applesauce mixture until all ingredients are thoroughly combined. Fold in the zucchini, apples, and walnuts.

Spray 2 loaf pans with vegetable spray. Divide the batter evenly among both pans. Bake at 350° for 55 minutes. Check for doneness by inserting a thin knife blade into the center. The knife blade will come out clean if the center is done. Dump the loaf onto a cooling rack and let cool until set enough to slice and serve warm.

Makes 2 loaves

Blueberry Coffee Cake

2	cups oat blend flour
1	teaspoon baking soda
2	teaspoons baking powder
½	teaspoon salt
4	tablespoons olive oil
¾	cup light brown sugar
1	egg
½	cup buttermilk
2	cups fresh blueberries, rinsed and drained

CRUMB TOPPING:

4	tablespoons butter
¼	cup oat flour
½	cup light brown sugar
½	teaspoon cinnamon

In a medium bowl sift together the flour, baking soda, baking powder, and salt. Set aside.

In a large bowl blend the oil and sugar together. Add the egg and buttermilk to the sugar mixture. Blend in the dry ingredients. Fold in the blueberries. Pour the batter into an oiled and floured 9-inch square baking dish.

Prepare the topping: In a small bowl blend the butter into the flour, sugar, and cinnamon with a pastry cutter. Sprinkle the crumb mixture over the surface. Bake at 375° for 40 to 45 minutes.

Serves 8

THIS RECIPE

is LOW in HEME iron and contains the following substances that inhibit absorption of nonheme iron:

✓ calcium

✓ dairy phosphate

✓ eggs

✓ phytate phosphorus

POLYPHENOLS

✓ tannic acid

chlorogenic acid

phenolic acid

oxalates

PER SERVING

IRON	heme iron	nonheme iron
	0.0 mg	0.76 mg

Bran Muffins

1¼ cups Nabisco brand bite-size shredded wheat with bran
1 cup brewed hot coffee
1 cup oat blend flour
2½ teaspoons baking soda
½ teaspoon salt
½ cup brown sugar
2 eggs, lightly beaten
½ cup applesauce
½ cup Faux Molasses (see page 258)
½ cup buttermilk
1 cup chopped English walnuts

THIS RECIPE

is LOW in HEME iron and contains the following substances that inhibit absorption of nonheme iron:

✓ calcium

✓ dairy phosphate

✓ eggs

✓ phytate phosphorus

POLYPHENOLS

✓ tannic acid

✓ chlorogenic acid

✓ phenolic acid

oxalates

PER SERVING

IRON	heme iron	nonheme iron
	0.0 mg	1.0 mg

Preheat the oven to 375°. Spray a 12-cup muffin pan with vegetable spray.

In a large bowl soak the cereal in coffee about 15 minutes.

In a separate bowl sift together the flour, soda, and salt. Set aside.

In a medium bowl mix the brown sugar and eggs together. Add the applesauce and faux molasses to the egg-sugar mixture, and blend well. Add to the cereal and mix well. Alternate adding milk and flour to the cereal mixture. Fold in the nuts. Scoop enough batter into each muffin cup to fill about two-thirds full. Bake for 17 minutes or until done.

Cool and refrigerate any remaining muffins. Warm in the microwave for 20 to 30 seconds before serving.

Makes 12

Buttermilk Biscuits

1½ cups oat blend flour
½ teaspoon salt
¼ teaspoon baking soda
½ teaspoon baking powder
¼ cup Crisco brand shortening
1 cup buttermilk

THIS RECIPE

*is LOW in HEME iron and contains
the following substances that
inhibit absorption of nonheme iron:*

✓ calcium

✓ dairy phosphate

eggs

✓ phytate phosphorus

POLYPHENOLS

tannic acid

chlorogenic acid

phenolic acid

oxalates

PER SERVING

IRON	heme iron	nonheme iron
	0.0 mg	0.3 mg

In a medium bowl sift the flour, salt, baking soda, and baking powder together and pile onto a pastry cloth. Cut the shortening into the flour until blended. Shape the dough into a pile. Make a well in the center. Slowly pour the buttermilk into the center, blending the edges from the outside into the milk. Continue adding milk and blending flour. The dough will be wet.

Preheat oven to 450°. Flour a rolling pin and roll out the dough very gently until about 1½ inches thick. Flour a biscuit cutter (the rim of a sturdy small glass can be used as a cutter) and cut out biscuits. Place close together in a shallow, ungreased baking dish. Bake at 450° for about 8 to 10 minutes until golden brown on top.

Serves 8

Coffee-Can Pumpkin Bread

3   cups oat blend flour
2   teaspoons baking soda
1   teaspoon salt
1   teaspoon nutmeg
1   teaspoon cinnamon
1/2 teaspoon ground cloves
2   cups light brown sugar
2/3 cup olive oil
2/3 cup buttermilk
1   egg
1   29-ounce can pumpkin
1/2 cup chopped English walnuts

THIS RECIPE

is LOW in HEME iron and contains the following substances that inhibit absorption of nonheme iron:

✓ calcium

✓ dairy phosphate

✓ eggs

✓ phytate phosphorus

POLYPHENOLS

✓ tannic acid

✓ chlorogenic acid

✓ phenolic acid

oxalates

PER SERVING

IRON	heme iron	nonheme iron
	0.0 mg	0.9 mg

Preheat the oven to 350°. Wash and completely dry four 1-pound coffee cans. Oil and flour the insides of cans. Set aside.

In a large bowl combine the flour, baking soda, salt, nutmeg, cinnamon, cloves, and brown sugar. Add the oil, buttermilk, egg, and pumpkin and mix well. Fold in the walnuts. Divide the batter equally among the 4 cans. Bake for 55 to 60 minutes. Check the center for doneness.

Allow to cool before removing the bread from the cans. Each should slip out easily; if not, slide a thin knife blade between the inside of the can and the bread.

Remove, cool further, wrap, and refrigerate.

Makes 4 "loaves"

Corn Bread

¼ cup olive oil
1 cup Yelton's brand cornmeal
1 cup oat blend flour
4 teaspoons baking powder
1 teaspoon baking soda
½ teaspoon salt
1 egg
1½ cups buttermilk

THIS RECIPE

*is LOW in HEME iron and contains
the following substances that
inhibit absorption of nonheme iron:*

✓ calcium

✓ dairy phosphate

✓ eggs

✓ phytate phosphorus

POLYPHENOLS

tannic acid

chlorogenic acid

phenolic acid

oxalates

PER SERVING

IRON	heme iron	nonheme iron
	0.0 mg	0.4 mg

Pour the oil in an 8-inch square glass baking dish. Heat the oil in a 450° oven.

In a medium bowl mix the cornmeal, flour, baking powder, baking soda, and salt. In a separate bowl mix the egg and buttermilk. Add the dry ingredients to the buttermilk mixture. When completely blended add the hot oil to the mixture. Stir and pour the batter into the heated baking dish. Bake for 15 minutes.

Serves 6 to 8

Dill Weed Bread

2½ cups whole-wheat flour
2 tablespoons sugar
1 teaspoon salt
¼ teaspoon baking soda
1 package dry yeast
¼ cup warm coffee
1 tablespoon olive oil
1 egg
1 cup buttermilk
2 tablespoons dill
1 tablespoon instant onion

THIS RECIPE

is LOW in HEME iron and contains the following substances that inhibit absorption of nonheme iron:

✓ calcium
✓ dairy phosphate
✓ eggs
✓ phytate phosphorus
POLYPHENOLS
✓ tannic acid
✓ chlorogenic acid
phenolic acid
✓ oxalates

PER SERVING

IRON	heme iron	nonheme iron
	0.0 mg	0.6 mg

In a medium bowl sift together the flour, sugar, salt, and baking soda.

In a large bowl soften the yeast with the warm coffee. Add the oil.

In a medium bowl lightly beat the egg, and add the buttermilk. Add the dill and onion.

Alternately add the dry ingredients and buttermilk mixture to the coffee mixture. The dough will become stiff. Turn out onto a pastry cloth and knead. Place in a large greased glass bowl. Cover with a tea towel and allow to rise until doubled in size, about 1 hour.

Turn out onto a pastry cloth. Punch down, knead, and divide into 2 loaves. Place in 2 well-greased and floured loaf pans. Cover and allow to rise for 45 minutes.

Bake at 350° for 45 to 50 minutes.

Makes 2 loaves (about 20 slices)

Herb Wheat Rolls

1	cup warm coffee
2	packages dry yeast
2	cups scalded lowfat milk
7¼	cups whole-wheat flour
2	teaspoons salt
½	teaspoon dried basil
½	teaspoon dried rosemary
½	teaspoon dried marjoram
½	teaspoon dried oregano
½	cup olive oil
2	eggs, lightly beaten

In a large bowl pour the warm coffee over the yeast.

Pour the scalded milk in a separate bowl and add a small amount of flour (about 1 cup). Stir in the salt, herbs, and oil. Then add the yeast-coffee mixture. Add flour slowly, then eggs, until all is combined. The dough will no longer stick to the edges of the bowl when properly combined. Turn the dough out onto a floured pastry cloth and let stand for 10 minutes.

Knead until elastic and smooth. Lightly oil the sides of a large bowl. Place the dough in a bowl, and cover with a tea towel. Let rise until doubled in size, about 1 hour.

Punch down, and shape into rolls. Allow to rise again for about 40 minutes.

Bake at 425° for about 10 to 12 minutes until the tops are golden brown.

Makes 36 rolls

THIS RECIPE

is LOW in HEME iron and contains the following substances that inhibit absorption of nonheme iron:

✓ calcium

✓ dairy phosphate

✓ eggs

✓ phytate phosphorus

POLYPHENOLS

✓ tannic acid

✓ chlorogenic acid

phenolic acid

✓ oxalates

PER SERVING

IRON	heme iron	nonheme iron
	0.0 mg	0.8 mg

Onion-Herb Corn Bread

¼ cup olive oil
2 tablespoons finely chopped onion
1 cup Yelton's brand cornmeal
1 cup oat blend flour
4 teaspoons baking powder
1 teaspoon baking soda
1 teaspoon dried basil
1 teaspoon dried oregano
½ teaspoon salt
1 egg
1½ cups buttermilk

THIS RECIPE

*is LOW in HEME iron and contains
the following substances that
inhibit absorption of nonheme iron:*

	✓ calcium
	✓ dairy phosphate
	✓ eggs
✓ phytate phosphorus	
POLYPHENOLS	
tannic acid	
chlorogenic acid	
phenolic acid	
	✓ oxalates

PER SERVING

IRON	heme iron	nonheme iron
	0.0 mg	0.4 mg

In a skillet heat the oil and sauté the onion until tender. Set aside.

In a medium bowl mix the cornmeal, flour, baking powder, baking soda, basil, oregano, and salt.

In a large bowl mix together the egg and buttermilk.

Pour the oil and onion in a glass baking dish. Heat in a 450° oven and heat for 5 to 7 minutes.

Meanwhile add the dry ingredients to the liquid mixture. When completely blended add the hot oil and onions to the batter. Stir and pour the batter into a heated baking dish. Bake for 15 minutes.

Serves 6 to 8

Peanut Butter Banana Muffins

1   cup whole-wheat flour
³/₄   cup Quaker brand oats
1   tablespoon baking powder
1   teaspoon baking soda
½   teaspoon salt
½   cup brown sugar
½   cup Jif brand peanut butter
1   banana, well mashed
1   tablespoon apple juice
1   teaspoon vanilla extract
2   tablespoons olive oil
1   egg
1   cup buttermilk

TOPPING:
¼   cup oats
¼   cup wheat flour
2   tablespoons butter, melted
2   tablespoons brown sugar

Spray a 12-cup muffin pan generously with vegetable spray. In a medium bowl sift together the flour, oats, baking powder, baking soda, and salt.

In a large bowl mix together the brown sugar, peanut butter, banana, apple juice, vanilla, and oil. Blend the egg and buttermilk, and add to the sugar mixture. Add the dry ingredients and mix just until moistened. Pour the batter evenly into the muffin pan.

In a small bowl combine the topping ingredients and mix until crumbly. Sprinkle the top of each muffin with the topping. Bake at 375° for 18 minutes.

Makes 12 muffins

THIS RECIPE

is LOW in HEME iron and contains the following substances that inhibit absorption of nonheme iron:

✓ calcium

✓ dairy phosphate

✓ eggs

✓ phytate phosphorus

POLYPHENOLS

✓ tannic acid

✓ chlorogenic acid

✓ phenolic acid

oxalates

PER SERVING

IRON	heme iron	nonheme iron
	0.0 mg	0.8 mg

Bean, Rice, and Cheese Wrap

½ cup Refried Beans (cooked according to recipe on page 68)

½ cup wild rice, cooked according to recipe with tea

½ cup shredded Cheddar cheese

2 soft tortillas (flour or corn)

4 fresh spinach leaves

¼ cup chopped spring onion (scallions)

THIS RECIPE

is LOW in HEME iron and contains the following substances that inhibit absorption of nonheme iron:

✓ calcium

✓ dairy phosphate

eggs

✓ phytate phosphorus

POLYPHENOLS

✓ tannic acid

chlorogenic acid

phenolic acid

✓ oxalates

PER SERVING

IRON	heme iron	nonheme iron
	0.0 mg	1.3 mg

In a medium bowl combine the beans, rice, and Cheddar cheese. Warm totillas by steaming them or covering in aluminum foil and baking in the oven on low heat.

Lay tortillas flat; spread the bean mixture down the center and sprinkle with spinach leaves and onion.

Fold two sides of each tortilla toward the center and then roll the opposite direction.

Serves 2

Chicken Fajita

2 boneless, skinless chicken breasts, cut into narrow strips
¼ cup water
1 teaspoon instant tea
½ teaspoon red pepper
¼ teaspoon paprika
½ teaspoon salt
1 tablespoon olive oil
1 cup thinly sliced onion
½ cup each: thinly sliced green and red bell peppers
4 tortilla or pita pockets

In a stockpot simmer the chicken in water and tea until done and the meat begins to brown around the edges. Sprinkle with red pepper and salt. Remove the meat and set aside.

In a skillet heat the oil and sauté the onion for 15 minutes until tender. Add the green pepper and continue cooking until the pepper is tender. Add the meat to the pan with the pepper and onion. Heat through. Divide portions evenly to fill 4 warm tortillas or pita pockets.

Serves 4

THIS RECIPE

is LOW in HEME iron and contains the following substances that inhibit absorption of nonheme iron:

calcium
✓ dairy phosphate
eggs
✓ phytate phosphorus
POLYPHENOLS
✓ tannic acid
✓ chlorogenic acid
phenolic acid
oxalates

PER SERVING

IRON	heme iron	nonheme iron
	0.2 mg	0.9 mg

Cucumber Veggie Club

1   ounce Neufchâtel cheese
3   slices whole-wheat bread
4   to 5 slices cucumber
1   onion, thinly sliced
1   slice tomato
2   slices avocado
     Pinch alfalfa sprouts

Spread Neufchâtel onto 2 slices of bread. On one slice place cucumbers and onion. Stack the next slice of bread, which is spread with Neufchâtel. Layer with avocado, tomato, and sprouts. Top with the last piece of bread. Cut diagonally and secure with toothpicks.

Serves 1

THIS RECIPE

is LOW in HEME iron and contains the following substances that inhibit absorption of nonheme iron:

✓ calcium

✓ dairy phosphate

eggs

✓ phytate phosphorus

POLYPHENOLS

✓ tannic acid

chlorogenic acid

phenolic acid

✓ oxalates

PER SERVING

IRON	heme iron	nonheme iron
	0.0 mg	3.9 mg

Eggplant Pocket

2	tablespoons olive oil
½	cup chopped onion
½	cup chopped pepper
½	cup raw eggplant strips
	Pinch oregano
½	cup brewed tea
1	cup Marinara Sauce (see page 243)

In a skillet heat the oil and sauté the onion until tender. Add the pepper, eggplant, oregano, and tea, and simmer until tender. Add the marinara sauce and simmer uncovered for 20 minutes. Spoon the mixture into pita pockets. Serve warm.

Serves 2

THIS RECIPE

is LOW in HEME iron and contains the following substances that inhibit absorption of nonheme iron:

calcium

✓ dairy phosphate

eggs

✓ phytate phosphorus

POLYPHENOLS

✓ tannic acid

chlorogenic acid

phenolic acid

✓ oxalates

PER SERVING

IRON	heme iron	nonheme iron
	0.0 mg	0.5 mg

Ham with Salami and Mustard Sauce

4 tablespoons reduced-fat mayonnaise
1 tablespoon spicy mustard
2 pita pockets
1 ounce thinly sliced hard salami
2 ounces thinly sliced deli ham
2 ounces Swiss cheese, cut julienne style

In a small bowl mix the mayonnaise and mustard and place in a squeeze bottle. Stuff the pita pockets with meat and cheese and squirt the sauce into the pockets.

Serves 2

THIS RECIPE

is LOW in HEME iron and contains the following substances that inhibit absorption of nonheme iron:

✓ calcium

✓ dairy phosphate

eggs

✓ phytate phosphorus

POLYPHENOLS

tannic acid

chlorogenic acid

phenolic acid

oxalates

PER SERVING

IRON	heme iron	nonheme iron
	0.2 mg	0.5 mg

Hamburger with Cheese and Onion

2 ounces ground beef
2 ounces ground turkey
1 tablespoon olive oil
¼ cup finely chopped onions
¼ cup brewed tea
　 Salt and pepper
1 slice creamy havarti cheese
1 hamburger bun

THIS RECIPE

is LOW in HEME iron and contains the following substances that inhibit absorption of nonheme iron:

✓ calcium

✓ dairy phosphate

eggs

✓ phytate phosphorus

POLYPHENOLS

✓ tannic acid

chlorogenic acid

phenolic acid

oxalates

PER SERVING

IRON	heme iron	nonheme iron
	0.5 mg	3.4 mg

In a medium bowl mix the beef and turkey and form into a patty. In a small skillet heat the oil and sauté the onions. Add the meat and tea. Season with salt and pepper. Simmer until the liquid evaporates.

Place cheese on top of the meat and cover so the cheese will melt. Toast the hamburger bun and place the patty and onions on the bottom half of the bun. Add mustard and ketchup to the top bun as desired.

Note: By mixing beef with turkey, the iron content is reduced by nearly a milligram, creating a low heme iron version of a classic American favorite—the hamburger.

Serves 1

Hot Dogs Deluxe

2   turkey hot dogs, split lengthwise
¼   cup brewed tea
¼   cup hot dog chili sauce (see page 134)
1   side of ⅓ loaf of French bread
2   tablespoons reduced-fat mayonnaise
     Garlic powder
     Pinch finely chopped fresh parsley
1   teaspoon spicy mustard
1   teaspoon finely chopped onion
¼   cup coleslaw
1   teaspoon ketchup
2   slices Muenster cheese

In a skillet sear the hot dogs over high heat. Add the tea and simmer for 10 minutes. Remove the meat from the pan and set aside. In a saucepan warm the chili sauce.

Split the bread down the center and cover with mayonnaise. Sprinkle with garlic powder and parsley. Place under the broiler until toasted. Remove from the oven but leave the broiler on. Spread mustard onto the toasted surface. Place hot dogs cut side down on the bread. Top with chili sauce, onion, slaw, ketchup, and cheese. Place under the broiler long enough to melt the cheese.

Serves 1

This Recipe

is LOW in HEME iron and contains the following substances that inhibit absorption of nonheme iron:

✓ calcium

✓ dairy phosphate

eggs

✓ phytate phosphorus

POLYPHENOLS

✓ tannic acid

chlorogenic acid

phenolic acid

✓ oxalates

Per Serving

IRON	heme iron	nonheme iron
	0.4 mg	0.9 mg

Chili Dogs

CHILI SAUCE:

1	tablespoon olive oil
¼	cup finely chopped onion
1	pound ground turkey
1	teaspoon salt
½	teaspoon red pepper
1	teaspoon cumin
3	tablespoons tomato paste
3	tablespoons ketchup
½	cup hot coffee
8	turkey hot dogs
8	whole-wheat hot dog buns

In a skillet heat the oil and sauté the onion until tender. Add the ground turkey, seasonings, tomato paste, ketchup, and coffee. Simmer for 20 to 30 minutes.

Heat the hot dogs. Place on the buns and top with sauce.

Tip: Place the hot dog with bun and sauce on a tray in a warm oven (275°) for 10 minutes. This steams the bun and brings out the flavor of the chili sauce. Top with your choice of fresh chopped onions, kraut, mustard, and ketchup.

Serves 8

THIS RECIPE

is LOW in HEME iron and contains the following substances that inhibit absorption of nonheme iron:

calcium

dairy phosphate

eggs

phytate phosphorus

POLYPHENOLS

✓ tannic acid

chlorogenic acid

phenolic acid

oxalates

PER SERVING

IRON	heme iron	nonheme iron
	0.26 mg	0.5 mg

Omelet Sandwich

2   slices Canadian bacon
½   cup brewed tea
2   tablespoons olive oil
½   cup finely chopped onion
¼   cup chopped green pepper
¼   cup chopped fresh tomato
     Salt and pepper to taste
3   eggs, lightly beaten
½   cup Muenster Cheese
2   bagels, split and toasted

THIS RECIPE

*is LOW in HEME iron and contains
the following substances that
inhibit absorption of nonheme iron:*

✓ calcium

✓ dairy phosphate

✓ eggs

✓ phytate phosphorus

POLYPHENOLS

✓ tannic acid

chlorogenic acid

phenolic acid

oxalates

PER SERVING

IRON	heme iron	nonheme iron
	0.3 mg	0.6 mg

In a hot skillet sear the Canadian bacon. Add the tea and cook until the liquid evaporates. Remove the meat, cut into thin strips, and set aside.

Add oil to the pan and sauté the onion until tender. Add the pepper and tomato and simmer. Season with salt and pepper. Add the beaten eggs and ham, and cook until the eggs are solid. Sprinkle the cheese over the eggs, cover, and turn off the heat. Let stand for 4 to 5 minutes until the cheese melts. Divide the omelet in half and serve on toasted bagels. Can be served open-faced on one half of a toasted bagel.

Serves 2

Open-Faced Hot Ham and Cheese

1   slice rye bread with caraway
     seed, lightly toasted
1   thin slice tomato
1   cluster broccoli florets (steamed
     in microwave)
3   ounces shaved ham
¼   cup Cheese Sauce (see page 238)

Place the toast on a plate. Add the tomato slice, then broccoli, and pile the ham on top. Heat in the microwave for 1 minute. Cover with hot cheese sauce.

Serves 1

THIS RECIPE

is LOW in HEME iron and contains the following substances that inhibit absorption of nonheme iron:

✓ calcium

✓ dairy phosphate

eggs

✓ phytate phosphorus

POLYPHENOLS

✓ tannic acid

chlorogenic acid

phenolic acid

oxalates

PER SERVING

IRON	heme iron	nonheme iron
	0.25 mg	1.6 mg

Pimiento Cheese Spread on Rye

1   7-ounce jar pimientos, sliced and drained
8   ounces Neufchâtel cheese
10 ounces extra-sharp Cheddar cheese, shredded
⅛   teaspoon red pepper (about 6 or 7 shakes)

In a food processor place the pimiento, and pulse 3 to 4 times. Add the Neufchâtel and pulse until the pimiento is blended. Add the shredded Cheddar and blend. Season with red pepper.

Spread on rye bread and serve.

Makes 2 cups

THIS RECIPE

is LOW in HEME iron and contains the following substances that inhibit absorption of nonheme iron:

calcium

✓ dairy phosphate

eggs

✓ phytate phosphorus

POLYPHENOLS

✓ tannic acid

✓ chlorogenic acid

phenolic acid

oxalates

PER SERVING

IRON	heme iron	nonheme iron
	trace	1.8 mg

Sausage and Peppers

¼ cup olive oil
1 cup thinly sliced onion
½ cup julienne-cut strips green bell pepper
½ pound mild turkey sausage, cut into 2-inch pieces and split
½ pound hot Italian sausage, cut into 2-inch pieces and split
1 cup Marinara Sauce (see page 243)
2 loaves French bread

In a skillet heat the oil and sauté the onions and peppers until tender. Place the sausages meat side up under the oven broiler long enough to char. Add the sausages to the onions and peppers. Add the marinara sauce and simmer until heated through.

Split open the French bread. Fill with sausage, peppers, and onions.

Serves 4

THIS RECIPE

is LOW in HEME iron and contains the following substances that inhibit absorption of nonheme iron:

calcium

dairy phosphate

eggs

✓ phytate phosphorus

POLYPHENOLS

✓ tannic acid

chlorogenic acid

phenolic acid

oxalates

PER SERVING

IRON	heme iron	nonheme iron
	0.4 mg	0.7 mg

Beef BBQ

1   pound lean sirloin beef
1   cup of brewed green tea
1   recipe BBQ Sauce (pg. 236)

Cook beef in green tea in slow cooker all day. Pull cooked meat apart Cover with BBQ sauce.

Serve on toasted buns.

Serves 4 to 6

THIS RECIPE

is HIGH in HEME iron and contains the following substances that inhibit absorption of nonheme iron:

calcium

dairy phosphate

eggs

phytate phosphorus

POLYPHENOLS

✓ tannic acid

chlorogenic acid

phenolic acid

oxalates

PER SERVING

IRON	heme iron	nonheme iron
	1.2 mg	3.4 mg

Sloppy Joes

2 tablespoons olive oil
½ cup finely chopped onion
½ cup finely chopped green bell pepper
¼ cup finely chopped celery
1 pound ground turkey
1 teaspoon salt
½ teaspoon red pepper
1 teaspoon cumin
1 teaspoon minced garlic
3 tablespoons tomato paste
½ cup hot coffee
⅔ cup ketchup
8 whole-wheat hamburger buns

In a skillet heat the oil and sauté the onion, bell pepper, and celery until tender. Add the turkey, salt, red pepper, cumin, and garlic, and sauté until the turkey is done. Add the tomato paste, hot coffee, and ketchup. Simmer for 20 to 30 minutes. Serve on whole-wheat hamburger buns.

Serves 6

THIS RECIPE

is LOW in HEME iron and contains the following substances that inhibit absorption of nonheme iron:

calcium

dairy phosphate

eggs

phytate phosphorus

POLYPHENOLS

✓ tannic acid

chlorogenic acid

phenolic acid

oxalates

PER SERVING

IRON	heme iron	nonheme iron
	0.4 mg	0.6 mg

Tuna Bacon Melt

2/3   cup Tuna Salad (see page 109)
2   slices toasted rye bread
3   strips crisp bacon, crumbled
4   slices Swiss cheese, cut julienne
     style

Divide the tuna salad onto the rye toast. Cover with crumbled bacon and cheese. Place under the broiler to melt the cheese.

Serves 2

THIS RECIPE

is LOW in HEME iron and contains the following substances that inhibit absorption of nonheme iron:

✓ calcium

✓ dairy phosphate

eggs

✓ phytate phosphorus

POLYPHENOLS

✓ tannic acid

chlorogenic acid

phenolic acid

oxalates

PER SERVING

IRON	heme iron	nonheme iron
	0.3 mg	0.7 mg

Tuna Melt with Black Olives and Roasted Peppers

¼   cup red or green bell pepper strips
     Olive oil
½   toasted English muffin
1   serving (about ⅓ cup) Tuna Salad (see page 109)
2   tablespoons chopped black olives
1   ounce shredded sharp Cheddar cheese

Brush the pepper with olive oil and cut into slivers. Place on a baking sheet and roast under the broiler until slightly burnt at the edges.

Toast the English muffin half. Scoop tuna onto the muffin. Add black olives and peppers. Cover the top with cheese. Heat under the broiler until the cheese melts or heat in the microwave (take care; bread can get tough).

Serves 1

THIS RECIPE

is LOW in HEME iron and contains the following substances that inhibit absorption of nonheme iron:

✓ calcium

✓ dairy phosphate

eggs

✓ phytate phosphorus

POLYPHENOLS

✓ tannic acid

chlorogenic acid

phenolic acid

oxalates

PER SERVING

IRON	heme iron	nonheme iron
	0.6 mg	0.8 mg

Turkey Club

8   ounces fresh baked turkey breast
8   strips bacon
2   tablespoons mayonnaise
1   tablespoon spicy mustard
12 slices whole-wheat bread
4   slices deli ham
4   lettuce leaves
4   slices tomato

PER SERVING

IRON	heme iron	nonheme iron
	0.5 mg	1.4 mg

Bake the turkey breast for 1 hour. Wrap and cool in the refrigerator overnight.

In the microwave cook the bacon until crisp.

In a small bowl combine the mayonnaise and mustard.

Toast the bread. Spread 4 slices of toast with the mayonnaise and mustard sauce. Top with ham and 2 slices of bacon. Top each with another slice of toast. Spread with sauce. Layer 2 ounces of sliced turkey, then lettuce and tomato on each sandwich. Top each sandwich with a piece of toast. Slice each club on the diagonal (corner to corner), creating triangles. Secure each triangle with a toothpick.

Serves 4

Turkey Wrap
with Pepper Mayonnaise

½	cup mayonnaise
¼	teaspoon black pepper
4	soft pita pockets
12	ounces thinly sliced turkey breast
4	slices Swiss cheese
4	fresh spinach leaves
4	thin slices red onion

In a small bowl mix the mayonnaise with the black pepper. Spread on the pita pockets. Layer turkey, cheese, spinach, and onion, fold in half, and serve.

Serves 4

THIS RECIPE

is LOW in HEME iron and contains the following substances that inhibit absorption of nonheme iron:

✓ calcium

✓ dairy phosphate

eggs

✓ phytate phosphorus

POLYPHENOLS

✓ tannic acid

chlorogenic acid

phenolic acid

✓ oxalates

PER SERVING

IRON	heme iron	nonheme iron
	trace	0.6 mg

Veggie Pocket

1 cup chopped leaf lettuce
¼ cup chopped onion
¼ cup cucumbers, scored and sliced thin
2 tablespoons Italian dressing
4 pita pockets
½ cup shredded sharp Cheddar cheese

In a medium bowl toss the lettuce, onion, and cucumber with the dressing. Fill pita pockets with salad and add cheese.

Serves 4

This Recipe

is LOW in HEME iron and contains the following substances that inhibit absorption of nonheme iron:

✓ calcium

✓ dairy phosphate

eggs

✓ phytate phosphorus

polyphenols

tannic acid

chlorogenic acid

phenolic acid

oxalates

Per Serving

IRON	heme iron	nonheme iron
	0.0	0.6 mg

Welsh Rarebit

¼ cup olive oil
2 tablespoons flour
1½ cups milk
½ cup brewed tea
1 cup cubed Velveeta cheese
1 cup shredded sharp Cheddar cheese
2 tablespoons tomato paste
1 teaspoon Worcestershire sauce
½ pound deli ham, shredded

In a saucepan heat the oil. Whisk the flour into the hot oil. Add the milk and tea, and blend well. Add the Velveeta, and stir until melted. Add the Cheddar, tomato paste, and Worcestershire sauce, and heat through. Then add the meat and reheat.

Serve over toasted rye.

Serves 4

THIS RECIPE

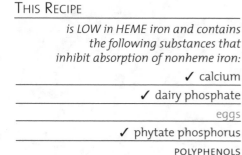

is LOW in HEME iron and contains the following substances that inhibit absorption of nonheme iron:

✓ calcium

✓ dairy phosphate

eggs

✓ phytate phosphorus

POLYPHENOLS

✓ tannic acid

chlorogenic acid

phenolic acid

oxalates

PER SERVING

IRON	heme iron	nonheme iron
	0.3 mg	0.8 mg

Healthy Single-Portion Pizza

1   sheet Streit's® Lightly Salted Matzos
10 turkey pepperoni slices
¼   cup low-sodium, no-sugar spaghetti sauce or tomato sauce (if using tomato sauce, add oregano, basil, and garlic to taste)
    Chopped onion
3   lowfat mozzarella sticks

THIS RECIPE

is LOW in HEME iron and contains the following substances that inhibit absorption of nonheme iron:

✓ calcium

dairy phosphate

eggs

phytate phosphorus

POLYPHENOLS

tannic acid

chlorogenic acid

phenolic acid

✓ oxalates

PER SERVING

IRON	heme iron	nonheme iron
	0.04 mg	1.4 mg

Preheat oven 425°.

Take about 10 pepperoni slices from the package and chop up very fine. Chop the onion very fine. Chop the mozzarella sticks by cutting lengthwise twice then chopping.

Take 1 whole Matzo from the box. Spread a thin layer (about ¼ cup) of sauce on the cracker. Sprinkle chopped pepperoni and onion over the sauce and top evenly with the finely chopped mozzarella pieces.

Bake in the oven until cheese is melted evenly and browned on top, about 15 mintues.

Serves 1

Recipe submitted by Adam Tanner

Barbecued Chicken

4   tablespoons olive oil
1   cup finely chopped onion
2   teaspoons minced garlic
1   small can tomato paste
2   cans hot strong black coffee
1   cup Heinz ketchup
¼   cup apple cider vinegar
½   cup brown sugar
2   tablespoons spicy mustard
½   teaspoon red pepper
4   7- to 8-ounce chicken breasts on the bone

In a saucepan heat the oil and sauté the onion and garlic until tender and golden, about 20 minutes.

Add the remaining ingredients except the chicken and simmer for 1 hour.

Refrigerate the sauce and use as needed.

Trim all excess fat from the chicken. Wash the chicken in cold water, pat dry, and place in glass cooking dish. Cover and bake at 350° for 1 hour.

Allow the meat to cool so the skin can be removed without burning fingers. Drain the broth and refrigerate for use in soup, rice, or sauces.

Once the skin is removed, generously cover the meat with barbecue sauce. Place the chicken under the broiler for 5 to 10 minutes until the barbecue sauce begins to char slightly. Remove and let stand for 10 minutes before serving.

Serves 4
Makes 4½ cups of sauce
Serving size: about 2 tablespoons

This Recipe

is LOW in HEME iron and contains the following substances that inhibit absorption of nonheme iron:

calcium

dairy phosphate

eggs

phytate phosphorus

POLYPHENOLS

✓ tannic acid

✓ chlorogenic acid

phenolic acid

oxalates

Per Serving

IRON	heme iron	nonheme iron
	0.4 mg	0.8 mg

Breaded Eggplant
with Pasta and Marinara Sauce

4   cups Marinara Sauce (see page 243)

     Pasta (linguini, angel hair, ziti, or your preference)

7   cups water
1   cup brewed tea
1   teaspoon salt
1   cup olive oil
1   medium eggplant with skin
2   cups flour for dredging
2   eggs, lightly beaten
2   cups bread crumbs
1   teaspoon salt
½   cup grated Parmesan cheese

THIS RECIPE

is LOW in HEME iron and contains the following substances that inhibit absorption of nonheme iron:

	✓ calcium
	✓ dairy phosphate
	✓ eggs
	✓ phytate phosphorus
	POLYPHENOLS
	✓ tannic acid
	✓ chlorogenic acid
	phenolic acid
	oxalates

PER SERVING

IRON	heme iron	nonheme iron
	0.0 mg	0.95 mg

Heat the marinara sauce and have ready to serve.

Prepare the pasta: In a large pot bring the water to a boil with the tea and 1 teaspoon of salt. Add the pasta and cook according to the time specified on the package.

In a skillet heat the olive oil on medium-high for frying. Wash, dry, and cut the eggplant first lengthwise then into medium width slices. Dredge first in flour, then in the eggs, then in bread crumbs. Drop in hot olive oil, brown, turn and brown the other side. Remove from the oil and place on a paper towel to drain. Sprinkle salt lightly over the surface of the fried eggplant.

On warm plates place the eggplant next to a serving of pasta, cover both with marinara, and top with Parmesan cheese.

Serves 4

Brunch Frittata

2 tablespoons olive oil
1/2 cup finely chopped yellow onion
1/2 teaspoon minced garlic
1 cup sliced mushrooms
1/2 cup chopped green pepper
1/2 cup ripe olives
5 eggs
1/3 cup light cream
1 teaspoon salt
1/8 teaspoon white pepper
1 8-ounce package Neufchâtel cheese, cut into small pieces
1 cup shredded Swiss cheese
1 1/3 cups torn rye bread

In a skillet heat the olive oil and sauté the onion and garlic. Add the mushrooms, green pepper, and olives.

In a medium bowl mix the eggs, cream, salt, white pepper, Neufchâtel cheese, and 1/2 cup of Swiss cheese. Spray a small square glass baking dish with vegetable spray. Line the bottom of the dish with bread. Slowly pour the mixture into the pan; stir to assure all ingredients are evenly distributed. Bake uncovered at 350° for 45 to 50 minutes. Let stand 10 minutes before serving.

Serves 6 to 8

THIS RECIPE

is LOW in HEME iron and contains the following substances that inhibit absorption of nonheme iron:

✓ calcium
✓ dairy phosphate
✓ eggs
✓ phytate phosphorus
POLYPHENOLS
✓ tannic acid
✓ chlorogenic acid
phenolic acid
oxalates

PER SERVING

IRON	heme iron	nonheme iron
	trace	1.2 mg

Buckwheat Pancakes with Spiced Apples and Coffee Syrup (Faux Molasses)

SPICED APPLES:

2	cups chopped apples
1/4	cup apple juice
1	teaspoon cinnamon
2	cups Faux Molasses (see page 258)

BUCKWHEAT PANCAKES:

2	tablespoons olive oil
1½	cups buckwheat flour
1½	teaspoons baking powder
1	teaspoon baking soda
1	teaspoon salt
1	teaspoon instant coffee
1½	cups buttermilk
2	eggs, lightly beaten
1	teaspoon vanilla extract

THIS RECIPE

is LOW in HEME iron and contains the following substances that inhibit absorption of nonheme iron:

✓ calcium

✓ dairy phosphate

✓ eggs

✓ phytate phosphorus

POLYPHENOLS

✓ tannic acid

✓ chlorogenic acid

✓ phenolic acid

oxalates

PER SERVING

IRON	heme iron	nonheme iron
	trace	2.06 mg

Place the apples in a saucepan with the apple juice, cinnamon, and 1 cup of Faux Molasses. Simmer until done. Set aside.

In a glass skillet heat the oil to medium-high. Place in a flour sifter all dry ingredients: flour, baking powder, soda, salt, and coffee.

In a medium bowl mix the buttermilk, eggs, and vanilla. Sift the dry ingredients into the egg-milk mixture *(Tip: Put the batter into a large measuring cup with spout for ease in pouring.)* Pour 4 equal dollops of batter into the hot skillet. Leave ample room as the cakes will expand. When bubbles form in the center of each cake, flip over to brown the other side. Remove and place on a warm plate.

Repeat until all batter is used.

Serve the pancakes topped with apples and the remaining Faux Molasses.

Serves 4 to 6

The Hemochromatosis Cookbook

Carbonara

7 cups water
1 cup brewed tea
1 teaspoon salt
1 pound angel hair pasta
¼ cup olive oil
⅓ cup each: shredded fontina, havarti, Parmesan cheeses
4 strips crisp bacon, crumbled
1 teaspoon fresh chopped parsley

In a stockpot bring the water to a boil with the tea and salt. Add the pasta and cook according to the time specified on the package. Rinse, drain, and return to the warm pot. Toss with olive oil. Add the cheeses, toss, and add bacon and parsley.

Serves 4

THIS RECIPE

is LOW in HEME iron and contains the following substances that inhibit absorption of nonheme iron:

✓ calcium

✓ dairy phosphate

eggs

✓ phytate phosphorus

POLYPHENOLS

✓ tannic acid

✓ chlorogenic acid

phenolic acid

oxalates

PER SERVING

IRON	heme iron	nonheme iron
	0.2 mg	2.0 mg

Chicken Asparagus Casserole

3	to 4 chicken breasts with ribs
2	cups water
1	cup brewed tea
1	cup Chicken Velouté (see page 240)
1	cup sour cream
¼	cup mayonnaise
1	10-ounce box frozen chopped asparagus
1	cup wild rice
1	cup water
1	cup brewed strong black tea
½	teaspoon salt

In a stockpot simmer the chicken breasts with rib in 2 cups of water and 1 cup of tea for 45 minutes. Remove the chicken and cool. Use the broth to prepare the velouté while the chicken cools.

Prepare the velouté and add the sour cream and mayonnaise.

Thaw the asparagus but do not cook. Place in a glass baking dish. When the chicken is sufficiently cooled, remove the meat from the bone and tear into pieces. Layer on top of the asparagus. Pour the sauce over the layered chicken and spread evenly. Bake at 375° for 1 hour or until brown.

Meanwhile prepare the rice. In a stockpot bring the water to a boil with the tea and salt. Add the rice, reduce the heat, cover, and steam for 25 minutes.

Serve the casserole over rice.

Serves 4 to 6

THIS RECIPE

is LOW in HEME iron and contains the following substances that inhibit absorption of nonheme iron:

✓ calcium

✓ dairy phosphate

eggs

✓ phytate phosphorus

POLYPHENOLS

✓ tannic acid

✓ chlorogenic acid

phenolic acid

oxalates

PER SERVING

IRON	heme iron	nonheme iron
	0.2 mg	0.5 mg

Chicken Carbonara
with Noodles Verte

7 cups water
1 cup brewed tea
1 teaspoon salt
½ pound spinach noodles
4 tablespoons olive oil
3 boneless skinless chicken breasts, cut into strips
¼ cup chopped prosciutto (Italian ham)
1 cup sliced mushrooms
¼ cup dry white wine
4 tablespoons whole-wheat flour
1 teaspoon salt
¼ teaspoon white pepper
½ cup strong coffee
1 cup chicken broth
½ cup light cream
¼ cup grated Parmesan cheese

THIS RECIPE

is LOW in HEME iron and contains the following substances that inhibit absorption of nonheme iron:

✓ calcium
✓ dairy phosphate
✓ eggs
✓ phytate phosphorus
POLYPHENOLS
✓ tannic acid
✓ chlorogenic acid
phenolic acid
✓ oxalates

In a large pot bring the water to a boil with the tea and salt. Add the noodles and cook according to the time specified on the package.

In a skillet heat 2 tablespoons of oil and sauté the chicken until brown on the edges. Remove the chicken and set aside. To the drippings add the ham, mushrooms, and wine, and continue cooking until the wine evaporates. Remove the mushroom/ham mixture. Add 2 tablespoons of oil to the pan. Whisk in the flour, salt, and pepper. Slowly add the coffee and whisk until the paste thickens. Add the broth and whisk until the sauce thickens. Add the ham-mushroom mixture, then stir in the light cream. Pour the sauce over the noodles, place the chicken strips on top, and sprinkle with Parmesan cheese.

Serves 4

PER SERVING

IRON	heme iron	nonheme iron
	0.5 mg	1.3 mg

Chicken Pot Pie

2   chicken breasts, 1 leg, and 1 thigh
2   cups water
1   cup brewed strong black tea
1   teaspoon salt
4   tablespoons olive oil
½   cup finely chopped onion
½   cup finely chopped celery
½   cup sliced mushrooms
4   tablespoons flour
     Pastry for a 2-crust pie (or butter-milk biscuit dough)
½   cup spring peas
½   cup cooked carrots
     Black pepper to taste
½   cup sour cream

THIS RECIPE

is LOW in HEME iron and contains the following substances that inhibit absorption of nonheme iron:

✓ calcium
✓ dairy phosphate
eggs
✓ phytate phosphorus
POLYPHENOLS
✓ tannic acid
✓ chlorogenic acid
phenolic acid
oxalates

PER SERVING

IRON	heme iron	nonheme iron
	0.25 mg	2.8 mg

In a saucepan simmer the chicken in 2 cups of water with 1 cup of tea for 45 minutes.

Remove the meat from the broth and set aside until cool. When cool enough to touch, pull the chicken from the bone and tear into small pieces—do not cut up the meat. Add 1 tablespoon of salt to the broth; reserve for sauce.

In a stockpot heat 2 tablespoons of olive oil and sauté the onion until tender. Add the celery and cook until tender. Add the mushrooms and cook 10 more minutes.

In a glass saucepan heat 2 tablespoons of the olive oil. Sprinkle the flour into the oil and whisk until a paste forms. Gently pour some of the broth into the paste; whisk until the sauce thickens, then slowly continue to add the broth a bit at a time so the sauce remains thick. Add the onion, celery, and mushrooms.

Line a baking dish with piecrust. Place a layer of pulled chicken on top of the crust. Add the spring peas and carrots. Season with black pepper to taste. Pour 2 cups of sauce over the layers. Reserve the remaining sauce for creamy gravy. Place the remaining crust on top, pinch the edges shut, and pierce the top with a fork to allow hot air to vent. Bake at 400° to 425° until the top crust is brown, about 50 minutes.

Heat the remaining sauce to a gentle boil. Reduce the heat and stir in the sour cream. Sauce can be optional on each serving of pot pie.

Serves 6

The Hemochromatosis Cookbook

Chicken Cordon Bleu

4	boneless chicken breasts (4 ounces each)
½	pound Swiss cheese
4	slices prosciutto (Italian ham)
1	cup flour for dredging
2	eggs, lightly beaten
1	cup whole-wheat bread crumbs
1	cup olive oil

THIS RECIPE

is LOW in HEME iron and contains the following substances that inhibit absorption of nonheme iron:

✓ calcium

✓ dairy phosphate

✓ eggs

✓ phytate phosphorus

POLYPHENOLS

✓ tannic acid

✓ chlorogenic acid

phenolic acid

oxalates

PER SERVING

IRON	heme iron	nonheme iron
	0.5 mg	0.76 mg

Place the chicken between 2 sheets of waxed paper. Gently pound the chicken until flattened. Place 2 ounces of cheese and 1 slice of ham in the center of each piece of chicken. Fold the flaps to the center, then roll up. Dredge in flour, then in egg, and finally the bread crumbs.

In a skillet heat the oil. Make certain the oil is very hot. Fry the rolled and breaded chicken until lightly browned. Remove and drain on paper towels. Place seam side down in a shallow baking dish. Cover and bake at 350° for 40 minutes.

Serves 4

Chicken and Herbed Dumplings

2 cups flour

1 teaspoon baking powder

2 teaspoons salt

8 cups hot chicken broth

1 egg, lightly beaten

1 tablespoon fresh chopped parsley

1 teaspoon chives

¼ teaspoon thyme

¼ teaspoon oregano

¼ teaspoon white pepper

1 cup brewed strong black tea

1 cup Chicken Velouté (see page 240)

½ cup light cream

3 chicken breasts, boiled and meat pulled from bone

In a medium bowl sift together the flour, baking powder, and 1 teaspoon of the salt. Add 1 cup of hot broth, then add the lightly beaten egg (do this quickly or the egg will cook). Fold in the herbs and pepper. Place the dough on a floured pastry cloth and roll out until about ¼ inch thick.

In a stockpot bring the remaining broth, tea, and remaining 1 teaspoon of salt to a boil. Cut the dumplings into 2-inch squares and drop in boiling tea broth. The dumplings will float when done. Remove the dumplings and set aside.

Heat the velouté and add the cream. Stir in the chicken, and serve over the dumplings.

Serves 4

THIS RECIPE

is LOW in HEME iron and contains the following substances that inhibit absorption of nonheme iron:

✓ calcium

✓ dairy phosphate

✓ eggs

✓ phytate phosphorus

POLYPHENOLS

✓ tannic acid

✓ chlorogenic acid

phenolic acid

✓ oxalates

PER SERVING

IRON	heme iron	nonheme iron
	0.3 mg	0.8 mg

Cubed Steak

4   cubed beef steaks
2   cups brewed tea
4   tablespoons olive oil
     Flour for dredging
     Salt and pepper to taste

THIS RECIPE

is HIGH in HEME iron and contains the following substances that inhibit absorption of nonheme iron:

calcium

dairy phosphate

eggs

✓ phytate phosphorus

POLYPHENOLS

✓ tannic acid

✓ chlorogenic acid

phenolic acid

oxalates

PER SERVING

IRON	heme iron	nonheme iron
	1.4 mg	1.2 mg

Allow the meat to marinate overnight in the tea.

In a skillet heat the olive oil for frying. Dredge the meat in flour. Brown the meat on both sides. Lightly salt and pepper the meat. Lower the heat, cover, and continue cooking for 10 minutes. Cut off the heat but do not lift the lid, and steam the meat for another 40 minutes.

Note: Beef contains high amounts of heme iron. Enjoy this entrée with low-iron vegetables, such as steamed collard greens, sautéed zucchini, sliced cucumber and onion salad, and tea as a beverage.

Serves 4

Gumbo with Turkey Sausage

6   cups Gumbo (see page 242)
1½   pounds turkey sausage
1   cup broth
1   cup brewed tea
1   teaspoon salt
1   cup rice
½   cup chopped spring onions
3   cups cooked black or red beans
     (see page 216)

THIS RECIPE

*is LOW in HEME iron and contains
the following substances that
inhibit absorption of nonheme iron:*

✓ calcium

✓ dairy phosphate

eggs

✓ phytate phosphorus

POLYPHENOLS

✓ tannic acid

✓ chlorogenic acid

phenolic acid

oxalates

PER SERVING

IRON	heme iron	nonheme iron
	0.6 mg	0.67 mg

In a saucepan heat the gumbo on medium low. Cut the turkey sausage diagonally into 1-inch pieces; split in half. Place in a baking dish under the broiler until the meat is slightly burned. Remove from the oven and add to the gumbo.

In a large saucepan bring the broth, tea, and salt to a boil. Add the rice. Cover, reduce the heat, and steam for 25 minutes.

Heat the beans in the microwave.

In large bowls place rice, then beans, cover with gumbo and meat. Top with spring onions.

Serves 6

Ham with Mustard Sauce

1 pound ham steak, thickly sliced
1 cup strong coffee
2 tablespoons olive oil
4 tablespoons whole-wheat flour
6 tablespoons dry mustard
$\frac{1}{2}$ cup light cream

THIS RECIPE

*is LOW in HEME iron and contains
the following substances that
inhibit absorption of nonheme iron:*

✓ calcium
✓ dairy phosphate
eggs
✓ phytate phosphorus
POLYPHENOLS
✓ tannic acid
✓ chlorogenic acid
phenolic acid
oxalates

PER SERVING

IRON	heme iron	nonheme iron
	0.4 mg	0.6 mg

In a large skillet over medium-high heat sear the ham. Add $\frac{1}{2}$ cup of coffee and cool until the liquid evaporates. Remove the meat and set aside. Add olive oil to the pan. Whisk in the flour and mustard. When the paste browns, slowly add the remaining coffee. When the mixture thickens, slowly add the cream. Heat through. Serve the sauce over the meat.

Serves 4

Herb-Encrusted Chicken

4   chicken breasts with ribs, skin removed and fat trimmed
1   cup buttermilk
1   teaspoon each: marjoram, thyme, rosemary, dill, and garlic powder
½   teaspoon paprika
½   teaspoon salt
¼   teaspoon red pepper
¼   teaspoon sugar

In a large bowl soak the chicken in buttermilk meat side down.

In a small bowl combine all herbs, seasonings, and sugar. Coat each chicken breast with the herb mixture until all of the mixture is used. Cover and bake at 375° for 45 minutes.

Remove the cover, increase the oven temperature to 400°, and bake an additional 10 minutes.

Serves 4

THIS RECIPE

is LOW in HEME iron and contains the following substances that inhibit absorption of nonheme iron:

✓ calcium

✓ dairy phosphate

eggs

✓ phytate phosphorus

POLYPHENOLS

✓ tannic acid

✓ chlorogenic acid

phenolic acid

oxalates

PER SERVING

IRON	heme iron	nonheme iron
	0.4 mg	0.6 mg

Italian Chicken

1	whole chicken
4	cups Marinara Sauce (see page 243)
2	bay leaves
1	tablespoon oregano
1	pound pasta
7	cups water
1	cup brewed tea
1	teaspoon salt
$\frac{1}{2}$	cup Parmesan or Romano cheese

Rinse the chicken in cold water and place in a baking dish. Cover with marinara sauce. Add bay leaves and oregano. Cover and bake at 300° for 2 hours.

Uncover and let stand for 10 minutes. Prepare the pasta in boiling water with tea and salt according to the time specified on the package (angel hair 6 minutes, vermicelli 7, etc.). Rinse, drain, and set aside.

Remove the bay leaves and discard. Separate the chicken from the bones, cartilage, and fat. Return the chicken to the sauce. Dump the pasta into the chicken-marinara sauce, toss, and turn out on warm plates. Top with cheese.

Serves 6

THIS RECIPE

is LOW in HEME iron and contains the following substances that inhibit absorption of nonheme iron:

✓ calcium

✓ dairy phosphate

eggs

✓ phytate phosphorus

POLYPHENOLS

✓ tannic acid

✓ chlorogenic acid

phenolic acid

✓ oxalates

PER SERVING

IRON	heme iron	nonheme iron
	0.5 mg	1.9 mg

Layered Taco Salad

2 cups cooked black beans
1½ cups shredded Cheddar or Monterey Jack cheese
4 cups shredded iceberg lettuce
1 teaspoon salt
1 cup diced fresh tomatoes
¼ cup sliced pitted black olives
2 roasted, peeled, and chopped poblano peppers
¼ cup chopped green onions
1 cup avocado dip
½ teaspoon cumin
2 cups coarsely crushed tortilla chips

In the bottom of a glass casserole dish layer in order the beans, cheese, lettuce, (sprinkle salt over lettuce layer), tomatoes, olives, peppers, and onions.

In a medium bowl mix together the avocado dip and cumin. Spread the avocado mixture over the top of the layered salad. Cover the dish with film wrap and refrigerate overnight.

Serve the salad over crushed tortilla chips.

Serves 6

THIS RECIPE

is LOW in HEME iron and contains the following substances that inhibit absorption of nonheme iron:

✓ calcium

✓ dairy phosphate

eggs

✓ phytate phosphorus

POLYPHENOLS

✓ tannic acid

✓ chlorogenic acid

phenolic acid

oxalates

PER SERVING

IRON	heme iron	nonheme iron
	trace	2.2 mg

Marinated Chicken

1 cup strong brewed tea
¼ cup balsamic vinegar
1 tablespoon minced garlic
1 teaspoon oregano
4 boneless chicken breasts, skin and fat removed
1 tablespoon cornstarch
¼ teaspoon salt
¼ cup water

In a flat glass casserole dish combine the tea, vinegar, garlic, and oregano. Rinse and pat dry each piece of chicken and place in the marinade. Refrigerate overnight, turning the meat once.

Place the chicken under the broiler for 8 minutes per side. Pour the marinade into a skillet.

In a shaker container mix the cornstarch, salt, and water. Shake vigorously and pour into the boiling marinade. Cook until the sauce is the consistency of gravy. Drizzle the sauce over the broiled chicken.

Serves 4

This Recipe

is LOW in HEME iron and contains the following substances that inhibit absorption of nonheme iron:

calcium

dairy phosphate

eggs

phytate phosphorus

POLYPHENOLS

✓ tannic acid

chlorogenic acid

phenolic acid

✓ oxalates

Per Serving

IRON	heme iron	nonheme iron
	0.4 mg	0.6 mg

Marinated Flank Steak

MARINADE:

2	**cups hot strong coffee**
1/4	**cup honey**
1	**tablespoon ground ginger**
1	**tablespoon soy sauce**
1 1/2	**pounds flank steak**

THIS RECIPE

is HIGH in HEME iron and contains the following substances that inhibit absorption of nonheme iron:

calcium

dairy phosphate

eggs

phytate phosphorus

POLYPHENOLS

✓ tannic acid

✓ chlorogenic acid

phenolic acid

oxalates

PER SERVING

IRON	heme iron	nonheme iron
	1.1 mg	3.2 mg

In a flat glass casserole dish combine the coffee, honey, ginger, and soy sauce. Place the meat in the dish and marinate in the refrigerator for 24 hours.

Remove the meat from the marinade. Prepare a grill.

Grill the meat on each side for 5 minutes, or place under the broiler for 10 minutes. Let stand for 10 minutes before slicing.

Slice the meat on an angle in thin slices.

Note: Due to the high heme content of this recipe, drink tea and serve this entrée with low-iron vegetables such as 1/2 cup green beans (0.37) and 1/2 cup fried cabbage and onions (0.45).

Serves 4

The Hemochromatosis Cookbook

Meatballs and Perciatelli

2 pounds ground turkey
1 teaspoon garlic powder
¼ cup chopped parsley
1 teaspoon salt
1 teaspoon black pepper
1 cup dried bread crumbs
⅔ cup grated Parmesan or Romano cheese
4 eggs
¾ cup buttermilk
8 cups Marinara Sauce (see page 243)
2 quarts water
1 teaspoon tea
1 teaspoon salt
1 pound perciatelli (long, thin macaroni)

Place the meat in a mixing bowl and add the garlic powder, parsley, salt, pepper, bread crumbs, and cheese. Add the eggs and buttermilk. Work the mixture by hand until well blended (sides of the bowl will be clean). Shape the mixture into 24 balls. Place on a lightly oiled cookie sheet and bake at 350° for 10 minutes.

Remove, drain, and place in marinara sauce. Simmer for 30 to 40 minutes.

In a large pot boil the water, tea, and salt. Drop the noodles into boiling water and cook for 15 to 18 minutes. Drain and rinse.

Serve the meatballs and sauce over the perciatelli.

Makes 24 meatballs; serves 8

THIS RECIPE

is LOW in HEME iron and contains the following substances that inhibit absorption of nonheme iron:

✓ calcium

✓ dairy phosphate

✓ eggs

✓ phytate phosphorus

POLYPHENOLS

✓ tannic acid

✓ chlorogenic acid

phenolic acid

oxalates

PER SERVING

IRON	heme iron	nonheme iron
	0.4 mg	2.1 mg

Meat Loaf

1 egg
½ cup strong black cold coffee
¼ cup oatmeal
¼ cup whole-wheat bread crumbs
1 pound ground turkey
¼ cup finely chopped onion
½ teaspoon salt
¼ teaspoon pepper
⅓ cup ketchup

In a large bowl lightly beat the egg and add the coffee. Add the oatmeal and bread crumbs, and mix well. Add the remaining ingredients except ketchup, and combine well (the best way is by hand). Place in a glass loaf pan. Spread ketchup over the top. Cover and bake at 350° for 40 minutes.

Uncover and continue baking for 15 minutes. Let the meat loaf stand for 10 to 15 minutes before serving.

Serves 4

THIS RECIPE

is LOW in HEME iron and contains the following substances that inhibit absorption of nonheme iron:

✓ calcium
✓ dairy phosphate
✓ eggs
✓ phytate phosphorus
POLYPHENOLS
✓ tannic acid
✓ chlorogenic acid
phenolic acid
oxalates

PER SERVING

IRON	heme iron	nonheme iron
	0.4 mg	2.3 mg

Mixed Grill Stir-Fry

½ cup strong black tea
¼ cup teriyaki sauce
1 teaspoon honey
1 tablespoon ground ginger
⅓ pound raw shrimp, cleaned
⅓ pound sirloin steak strips
⅓ pound chicken breast strips
2 cups broth
1 teaspoon salt
1 cup rice
2 tablespoons cornstarch
1 tablespoon olive oil
1 pound fresh asparagus spears, ends snapped
1 yellow summer squash, cut into julienne strips
1 teaspoon fresh chives

THIS RECIPE

is LOW in HEME iron and contains the following substances that inhibit absorption of nonheme iron:

✓ calcium
✓ dairy phosphate
eggs
✓ phytate phosphorus
POLYPHENOLS
✓ tannic acid
✓ chlorogenic acid
phenolic acid
oxalates

PER SERVING

IRON	heme iron	nonheme iron
	0.6 mg	1.2 mg

In a shallow dish combine the tea, teriyaki, honey, and ginger. Add the shrimp, steak strips, and chicken strips, and marinate overnight in the refrigerator.

Prepare the rice. In a stockpot bring 2 cups of broth, 1 teaspoon of salt, and the rice to a boil. Cook according to the time specified on the rice package.

Reserve ¼ cup of the marinade. In a glass skillet bring the remaining marinade to a boil. Place the reserved ¼ cup of marinade and the cornstarch in a small container with a lid and shake vigorously. Slowly pour the cornstarch-marinade mixture into the boiling liquid. Whisk vigorously until the liquid thickens; set aside.

In a separate skillet heat the olive oil. Sear the meat in the oil until done, about 8 to 10 minutes. Do not overcook; shrimp can get tough and chewy. Transfer the meat to the teriyaki marinade sauce.

Steam the asparagus and squash on the stovetop or in the microwave. Sprinkle the vegetables with chopped fresh chives and serve with the meat.

Serves 4

Mushroom-Stuffed Pork Chops

4   6-ounce pork chops with pockets (butcher will cut pocket upon request)

1   cup strong black tea

½   cup dry white wine

3   tablespoons olive oil
    Flour for dredging

½   cup finely chopped onion

⅛   teaspoon thyme

1   teaspoon oregano

½   teaspoon black pepper

2   cups sliced mushrooms

½   cup light cream

THIS RECIPE

is LOW in HEME iron and contains the following substances that inhibit absorption of nonheme iron:

✓ calcium

✓ dairy phosphate

eggs

✓ phytate phosphorus

POLYPHENOLS

✓ tannic acid

✓ chlorogenic acid

phenolic acid

oxalates

PER SERVING

IRON	heme iron	nonheme iron
	0.4 mg	0.65 mg

Trim all visible fat from the chops. In a shallow dish combine the strong tea and white wine and marinate the pork chops overnight in the mixture.

In a glass skillet heat 2 tablespoons of the oil. Dredge the chops in flour and brown in the oil. Remove, drain, and set aside. Add the remaining 1 tablespoon of oil and sauté the onion. Add the thyme, oregano, and pepper, and cook until the onion is tender, about 10 minutes.

Add the mushrooms and ½ cup of the marinade. Cook down until the liquid has evaporated. Spoon the mushroom-herb mixture into the pocket. Retain the pan drippings. Place the pork chops in a glass baking dish, cover, and bake at 300° for 50 minutes. Add the drippings from the baking dish to the previous reserve of drippings in the skillet. Turn up the heat and whisk in 1 teaspoon of flour, then slowly add the remaining marinade. When thickened, add the light cream and heat through. Pour over the chops.

Serves 4

Oven Enchiladas

2	tablespoons olive oil
½	cup chopped onion
1	pound ground turkey
1	teaspoon cumin
1	teaspoon salt
¼	teaspoon black pepper
4	ounces cream cheese
8	corn tortillas
½	cup enchilada sauce
½	cup shredded Monterey Jack cheese
½	cup sliced black olives
	Jalapeño peppers (optional)

In a large skillet heat the olive oil and sauté the onion until tender. Add the meat and brown. Add the cumin, salt, and pepper. Add the cream cheese and stir until melted.

Wrap the tortillas in foil and warm in a preheated 300° oven.

Spoon the meat-cheese filling onto one end of each tortilla and roll up. Place seam side down in a shallow baking dish. Top with enchilada sauce, shredded Monterey Jack cheese, black olives, and jalapeño peppers. Cover and bake at 350° for 30 to 40 minutes.

Serves 6 to 8

THIS RECIPE

is LOW in HEME iron and contains the following substances that inhibit absorption of nonheme iron:

✓ calcium

✓ dairy phosphate

eggs

✓ phytate phosphorus

POLYPHENOLS

tannic acid

chlorogenic acid

phenolic acid

oxalates

PER SERVING

IRON	heme iron	nonheme iron
	0.7 mg	3.8 mg

Oven-Fried Catfish

4   catfish fillets
1   cup seedless rye bread crumbs
1   tablespoon whole-wheat flour
1   tablespoon chopped fresh parsley
¼   teaspoon paprika
     Pinch red pepper
2   tablespoons grated Parmesan cheese
1   cup buttermilk
     Nonstick vegetable spray

In a shallow dish combine the bread crumbs, flour, parsley, paprika, red pepper, and Parmesan cheese. Coat the fish with buttermilk, then dredge in bread crumb mixture.

Spray a glass baking dish with cooking spray. Place the catfish in the dish. Bake uncovered at 400° for about 20 minutes. Do not overcook; when the fish is done it will be flaky.

Serves 4

This Recipe

is LOW in HEME iron and contains the following substances that inhibit absorption of nonheme iron:

✓ calcium

✓ dairy phosphate

eggs

✓ phytate phosphorus

POLYPHENOLS

✓ tannic acid

✓ chlorogenic acid

phenolic acid

oxalates

Per Serving

IRON	heme iron	nonheme iron
	0.3 mg	1.4 mg

Oven-Fried Chicken

½ cup buttermilk
½ cup plain yogurt
4 chicken breasts with ribs, skin and visible fat removed
2 cups bread crumbs
1 teaspoon paprika
1 teaspoon onion powder
1 teaspoon garlic powder
1 teaspoon salt
½ teaspoon oregano
½ teaspoon basil
½ teaspoon pepper

In a shallow dish mix the buttermilk and yogurt together. Place the chicken meat side down in the mixture and soak for 1 hour.

In a separate shallow dish combine the bread crumbs and remaining ingredients. Coat the chicken in the bread crumb mixture.

Preheat the oven to 400°. Place the chicken meat side up on an ungreased baking sheet. Bake for 45 minutes.

Let the chicken stand for 10 to 15 minutes before serving.

Serves 4

This Recipe

is LOW in HEME iron and contains the following substances that inhibit absorption of nonheme iron:

✓ calcium
✓ dairy phosphate
eggs
✓ phytate phosphorus
POLYPHENOLS
✓ tannic acid
✓ chlorogenic acid
phenolic acid
oxalates

Per Serving

IRON	heme iron	nonheme iron
	0.4 mg	0.6 mg

Parsnips and Pork Roast

3 to 4 pounds pork roast, all fat trimmed
1 teaspoon rubbed sage
Oat blend flour for dredging
2 tablespoons olive oil
1 cup strong coffee
Salt to taste
1 bay leaf
1 teaspoon marjoram
½ pound parsnips, rinsed, ends trimmed

Rub the outside of the pork with sage and dredge in flour. In a skillet heat the oil and brown the roast. Place the roast in a large glass casserole with lid. Add the coffee, salt, bay leaf, and marjoram. Cover the roast and bake at 350° for 2½ hours.

Place parsnips around the roast and continue cooking for 15 minutes. Turn the oven off and let the roast and parsnips steam in the oven for 40 minutes. Remove the bay leaf before serving.

Serves 6 to 8

THIS RECIPE

is LOW in HEME iron and contains the following substances that inhibit absorption of nonheme iron:

calcium
✓ dairy phosphate
eggs
✓ phytate phosphorus
POLYPHENOLS
✓ tannic acid
chlorogenic acid
phenolic acid
✓ oxalates

PER SERVING

IRON	heme iron	nonheme iron
	0.68 mg	0.5 mg

The Hemochromatosis Cookbook

Pasta e Fagioli
(Macaroni and Bean Soup)

1   pound dried navy beans or other small white beans
4   quarts water
3   teaspoons salt
1   teaspoon instant tea
¼   cup olive oil
2   tablespoons minced garlic
1½   cups diced tomatoes
1   cup chicken broth
2   tablespoons chopped fresh parsley
1   teaspoon dried basil
1   pound elbow macaroni
1   cup brewed tea
½   cup Parmesan cheese
½   teaspoon freshly ground black pepper

THIS RECIPE

is LOW in HEME iron and contains the following substances that inhibit absorption of nonheme iron:

✓ calcium

✓ dairy phosphate

eggs

✓ phytate phosphorus

POLYPHENOLS

✓ tannic acid

✓ chlorogenic acid

phenolic acid

oxalates

PER SERVING

IRON	heme iron	nonheme iron
	0.0 mg	4.2 mg

Wash beans thoroughly, picking out rocks and dirt. In a large pot bring 2 quarts of water to a boil. Add the beans, 1 teaspoon of salt, and tea. Reduce the heat and simmer for 2 hours or until the beans are tender. Drain the beans and set aside.

In a separate stockpot heat the oil and sauté the garlic. Add the tomatoes, chicken broth, 1 teaspoon of salt, parsley, and basil, and simmer at least 20 to 30 minutes.

In a separate pot bring 2 quarts of water to a boil. Add the macaroni, 1 teaspoon of salt, and tea, and cook for 10 minutes. Drain and reserve some of the liquid.

Add the beans and macaroni to the tomato mixture. Adjust the consistency by mashing beans if the dish is too moist, or by adding beans or macaroni broth if too dry. Consistency should be thick (stew-like). Add Parmesan and black pepper.

Serves 8

Pepper Caraway Chicken

4 chicken breasts, skin and fat removed
1 cup buttermilk
½ cup rye bread crumbs with caraway
½ teaspoon salt
¼ cup coarse ground black pepper
2 tablespoons olive oil

THIS RECIPE

is LOW in HEME iron and contains the following substances that inhibit absorption of nonheme iron:

✓ calcium
✓ dairy phosphate
eggs
✓ phytate phosphorus
POLYPHENOLS
✓ tannic acid
✓ chlorogenic acid
phenolic acid
oxalates

PER SERVING

IRON	heme iron	nonheme iron
	0.4 mg	1.8 mg

Rinse the chicken in cold water and pat dry. Place in buttermilk meat side down.

In a shallow dish mix the bread crumbs, salt, and pepper. Dredge the chicken in the crumb mixture, making certain each piece of meat is well coated and the pepper is evenly distributed.

In a skillet heat the oil over medium-high heat. Place the chicken meat side down in the hot oil, reduce the heat to medium, and brown the meat for about 15 to 20 minutes.

Cover the chicken, cut off the heat, and let slow cook for 40 to 45 minutes.

Serves 4

Pork Chops with Barbecued Peppers and Onions

3   tablespoons olive oil
4   medium-thick center cut pork chops
1   cup flour for dredging
½   cup barbecue sauce
1   cup green pepper strips (julienne style)
1   cup finely chopped onion

In a glass skillet heat 2 tablespoons of olive oil. Lightly coat the chops in flour. Brown the meat on one side, then the other. Remove and place in a shallow baking dish. Cover and bake at 350° for 1 hour.

In a saucepan heat the barbecue sauce.

In a clean skillet heat the remaining tablespoon of oil and sauté the onion and green pepper. Stir the barbecue sauce into the pepper and onion. Serve the sauce over the meat.

Serves 4

THIS RECIPE

is LOW in HEME iron and contains the following substances that inhibit absorption of nonheme iron:

calcium

✓ dairy phosphate

eggs

✓ phytate phosphorus

POLYPHENOLS

✓ tannic acid

✓ chlorogenic acid

phenolic acid

oxalates

PER SERVING

IRON	heme iron	nonheme iron
	0.4 mg	1.4 mg

Pork Marsala

1 pound pork tenderloin, sliced into ¼-inch-thick pieces
¼ cup flour
¼ cup olive oil
¼ cup dry white wine
1 cup sliced mushrooms
2 teaspoons salt
¼ cup apple juice
7 cups water
1 cup brewed strong black tea
1 teaspoon salt
12 ounces spinach noodles

THIS RECIPE

is LOW in HEME iron and contains the following substances that inhibit absorption of nonheme iron:

✓ calcium

✓ dairy phosphate

eggs

✓ phytate phosphorus

POLYPHENOLS

✓ tannic acid

✓ chlorogenic acid

✓ phenolic acid

oxalates

PER SERVING

IRON	heme iron	nonheme iron
	0.4 mg	1.9 mg

Dredge the meat in flour. In a skillet heat the oil and brown the tenderloin slices. Set aside.

Add the apple juice to the drippings. Add the mushrooms and cook until the liquid evaporates. Add 1 teaspoon of salt and the wine. Replace the meat, cover, and simmer on very low heat for 30 minutes.

In a stockpot bring the water to a boil with the tea and salt, and drop in the noodles. Boil for 7 to 8 minutes or according to the time specified on the package. Drain and rinse; if necessary reheat in the microwave or oven.

Serve the meat and mushrooms over the noodles.

Note: The alcohol content is lost during cooking.

Serves 6

Pork Tetrazzini

1	pound lean pork, cut into strips
	Flour for dredging
4	tablespoons olive oil
4	tablespoons flour
1	teaspoon salt
1/4	teaspoon white pepper
1/2	cup dry white wine
1	cup chicken broth
1	cup brewed tea
1/8	teaspoon ground thyme
7	cups water
1	cup brewed tea
1	teaspoon salt
1/2	pound spaghetti
1/2	cup grated Parmesan cheese

Dredge the pork strips in flour. In a skillet heat 2 tablespoons of olive oil and brown the meat. Set aside.

To the pan drippings add the remaining 2 tablespoons of oil. Whisk in the flour, thyme, salt, and pepper until smooth. Add the wine. Slowly add the broth and 1 cup of tea and whisk until thickened.

In a stockpot bring the water to a boil and add 1 cup of tea and the salt. Add the spaghetti and boil for the length of time suggested on the package. Drain, rinse, and pour into a casserole dish sprayed with vegetable spray. Layer the meat over the spaghetti and cover with sauce. Top with Parmesan cheese. Bake at 350° for 45 minutes.

Serves 6

THIS RECIPE

is LOW in HEME iron and contains the following substances that inhibit absorption of nonheme iron:

calcium

✓ dairy phosphate

eggs

✓ phytate phosphorus

POLYPHENOLS

✓ tannic acid

✓ chlorogenic acid

phenolic acid

oxalates

PER SERVING

IRON	heme iron	nonheme iron
	0.5 mg	2.1 mg

Roasted Chicken
with Vegetables and Rice

1   cup water
1   cup brewed tea
1   teaspoon salt
1   cup basmati rice
½   cup chopped fresh spinach
½   cup diced fresh tomatoes
     Red pepper to taste
1   small whole chicken, excluding
     organ meats
1   teaspoon salt

In a deep casserole dish place 1 cup of water and the tea. Add the salt, rice, spinach, tomatoes, and red pepper.

Rinse the chicken completely in cold water. Place the chicken in the casserole dish over the rice mixture. Cover and bake at 400° for 30 minutes.

Reduce the heat to 300° and continue cooking for 1 hour.

Remove the dish from the oven, uncover, and let stand for 10 to 15 minutes.

Serves 4

THIS RECIPE

*is LOW in HEME iron and contains
the following substances that
inhibit absorption of nonheme iron:*

✓ calcium

✓ dairy phosphate

eggs

✓ phytate phosphorus

POLYPHENOLS

✓ tannic acid

✓ chlorogenic acid

phenolic acid

✓ oxalates

PER SERVING

IRON	heme iron	nonheme iron
	0.6 mg	1.9 mg

Salmon Patties
with Horseradish Sauce

HORSERADISH SAUCE:

1½	cups sour cream
2	tablespoons horseradish
1	teaspoon lemon juice
6	dashes red pepper sauce
	Salt to taste

SALMON PATTIES:

1	10-ounce can salmon, drained (bones optional)
1	egg
2	tablespoons chopped fresh parsley
	Pinch red pepper
1	cup ground saltine crackers
½	cup olive oil for frying

In a small bowl combine all of the Horseradish Sauce ingredients and mix well.

In a medium bowl combine the salmon, egg, parsley, red pepper, and ½ cup of cracker crumbs. Form into patties and press into the remaining crumbs.

In a skillet heat the oil and fry the salmon patties until golden brown and crisp. Turn over and fry the other side until crisp. Remove and drain. Serve hot with Horseradish Sauce on the side.

Serves 6

THIS RECIPE

is LOW in HEME iron and contains the following substances that inhibit absorption of nonheme iron:

✓ calcium

✓ dairy phosphate

✓ eggs

✓ phytate phosphorus

POLYPHENOLS

tannic acid

chlorogenic acid

phenolic acid

oxalates

PER SERVING

IRON	heme iron	nonheme iron
	0.4 mg	1.1 mg

Sausage and Three-Cheese Breakfast Casserole

4	slices rye bread with caraway seed
4	eggs, lightly beaten
1	cup 1% milk
2	tablespoons olive oil
¼	cup finely chopped onion
1	teaspoon chopped fresh parsley
1	pound turkey sausage
½	cup sliced mushrooms
½	teaspoon salt
	Pinch red pepper
½	cup shredded Vermont or New York sharp white Cheddar
½	cup cubed Swiss cheese
½	cup fontina cheese

Arrange the slices of bread in the bottom of a shallow glass baking dish.

In a medium bowl mix the eggs and milk together and pour over the bread. Cover and refrigerate overnight.

In a skillet heat the olive oil and sauté the onion until tender. Add the parsley, then the sausage, and cook until the meat is done. Add the mushrooms, salt, and red pepper, and cook until the liquid has evaporated.

Layer the meat mixture over the soaked bread and cover with cheeses. Bake uncovered at 350° for 40 minutes.

Let stand for 10 minutes before serving.

Serves 6

THIS RECIPE

is LOW in HEME iron and contains the following substances that inhibit absorption of nonheme iron:

✓ calcium

✓ dairy phosphate

✓ eggs

✓ phytate phosphorus

POLYPHENOLS

tannic acid

chlorogenic acid

phenolic acid

oxalates

PER SERVING

IRON	heme iron	nonheme iron
	0.4 mg	1.5 mg

Seafood Casserole

1/4 cup olive oil

2 tablespoons whole-wheat flour

1 teaspoon salt

1/4 teaspoon white pepper

1/2 cup lowfat milk

1/2 teaspoon Worcestershire sauce

1/4 cup dry white wine

1 cup grated Swiss cheese

1/2 cup light cream

1 cup crushed saltine crackers

2/3 pound fresh flounder fillets

1/3 pound small shrimp, cleaned and deveined

1 tablespoon chives

In a saucepan heat the olive oil. Whisk in the flour, salt, and pepper. Slowly pour in the milk, whisk, and allow to thicken. Add the Worcestershire sauce and wine, and blend well. Add 2/3 cup of Swiss cheese and stir until melted. Drizzle in the cream and heat through, but do not boil.

Spray a glass casserole dish with vegetable spray. Spread crackers over the bottom of the dish. Arrange the fillets on top of the crackers. Spread shrimp evenly over the fillets. Cover the fish with sauce, sprinkle with chives, and top with the remaining cheese. Bake uncovered at 350° for 45 minutes.

Serves 6

THIS RECIPE

is LOW in HEME iron and contains the following substances that inhibit absorption of nonheme iron:

✓ calcium

✓ dairy phosphate

eggs

✓ phytate phosphorus

POLYPHENOLS

tannic acid

chlorogenic acid

phenolic acid

oxalates

PER SERVING

IRON	heme iron	nonheme iron
	0.2 mg	1.96 mg

Seafood Lasagna

3   quarts water
1   tablespoon instant tea
1   teaspoon salt
1   pound lasagna
1   cup ricotta cheese
½   cup finely chopped cooked fresh spinach
1   egg
     Leftover fish/shrimp from seafood stock
1   cup mozzarella cheese
½   cup grated Parmesan cheese

EASY ALFREDO SAUCE:
1½   cups sour cream
½   cup grated Parmesan cheese

In a stockpot boil the water, salt, and tea. Drop the lasagna noodles into the boiling water, set a timer, and boil for 6 minutes. Drain, rinse, and set aside the noodles.

In a mixing bowl combine the ricotta, spinach, egg, and fish. Alternate layers of spinach mixture, then mozzarella and Parmesan, ending with cheese. Bake uncovered at 350° for 45 minutes to 1 hour.

Let stand for 15 minutes before serving.

In a small bowl combine the sour cream and Parmesan cheese. Serve the Easy Alfredo Sauce over the top of the lasagna.

Serves 6

THIS RECIPE

is LOW in HEME iron and contains the following substances that inhibit absorption of nonheme iron:

✓ calcium

✓ dairy phosphate

✓ eggs

phytate phosphorus

POLYPHENOLS

✓ tannic acid

chlorogenic acid

phenolic acid

✓ oxalates

PER SERVING

IRON	heme iron	nonheme iron
	0.4 mg	2.8 mg

Sesame Chicken

1   cup buttermilk
½   cup apple juice
2   cloves garlic, peeled and smashed
4   tablespoons Greek seasoning
1   pound boneless, skinless chicken breasts
2   cups bread crumbs
½   cup sesame seeds
1   6-ounce jar plum jam
1   tablespoon fresh horseradish
1   teaspoon spicy mustard
1   tablespoon apple juice

In a shallow dish combine the buttermilk, apple juice, garlic, and Greek seasonings. Soak the chicken in the mixture overnight.

Remove the chicken and dredge in bread crumbs, then sesame seeds. Spray a cookie sheet with vegetable spray. Bake at 400° for about 20 minutes or until golden brown.

In a saucepan combine the plum jam, horseradish, mustard, and apple juice, mix well, and heat through.

Serve the chicken with the mustard plum sauce.

Serves 6

THIS RECIPE

is LOW in HEME iron and contains the following substances that inhibit absorption of nonheme iron:

calcium
✓ dairy phosphate
eggs
phytate phosphorus
POLYPHENOLS
✓ tannic acid
chlorogenic acid
phenolic acid
oxalates

PER SERVING

IRON	heme iron	nonheme iron
	0.4 mg	3.7 mg

Shrimp Creole

2 tablespoons olive oil

1 cup finely chopped onion

2 stalks celery, strings removed and cut in $\frac{1}{2}$-inch pieces

1 green pepper, seeded and sliced in strips

1 28-ounce can crushed tomatoes with sauce

1 6-ounce can tomato paste

3 cans hot brewed tea ($2\frac{1}{4}$ cups)

1 teaspoon dried basil

1 teaspoon dried thyme

$\frac{1}{4}$ to $\frac{1}{2}$ teaspoon red pepper (depends on personal taste for spiciness)

1 pound shrimp, peeled and de-veined (pat dry between paper towels)

$2\frac{1}{2}$ cups cooked wild rice

In a stockpot heat the oil and sauté the onions for 15 to 20 minutes until tender. Add the celery and green pepper, and simmer for 5 to 7 minutes.

Add the tomatoes, paste, and hot tea, and mix well. Add the basil, thyme, and pepper. Add the raw shrimp. Bring to a boil and cook until the shrimp curl.

Serve the shrimp and sauce over rice.

Serves 6

THIS RECIPE

is LOW in HEME iron and contains the following substances that inhibit absorption of nonheme iron:

calcium

dairy phosphate

eggs

phytate phosphorus

POLYPHENOLS

✓ tannic acid

chlorogenic acid

phenolic acid

oxalates

PER SERVING

IRON	heme iron	nonheme iron
	0.5 mg	4.56 mg

The Hemochromatosis Cookbook

Spaghetti with Meat Sauce

½ pound ground turkey
¼ cup coffee
8 cups Marinara Sauce (see page 243)
2 quarts water
1 teaspoon salt
1 teaspoon instant tea
1 pound spaghetti of choice
   Parmesan cheese for topping

In a saucepan cook the turkey in the coffee until done. Add the marinara sauce and simmer for 20 to 30 minutes.

In a stockpot bring the water, salt, and tea to a boil. Drop the pasta into the boiling water and stir well. When done, drain and rinse the pasta.

Top with sauce and warm in the microwave.

Sprinkle Parmesan cheese over the sauce.

Serves 4

THIS RECIPE

is LOW in HEME iron and contains the following substances that inhibit absorption of nonheme iron:

calcium

dairy phosphate

eggs

phytate phosphorus

POLYPHENOLS

✓ tannic acid

chlorogenic acid

phenolic acid

oxalates

PER SERVING

IRON	heme iron	nonheme iron
	0.3 mg	3.2 mg

Spinach Lasagna

1 cup cooked fresh spinach, drained
24 lasagna noodles
2 eggs
1 cup ricotta cheese
4 cups Marinara Sauce (see page 243)
2 cups mozzarella cheese
½ cup Parmesan cheese

THIS RECIPE

is LOW in HEME iron and contains the following substances that inhibit absorption of nonheme iron:

✓ calcium

✓ dairy phosphate

eggs

phytate phosphorus

POLYPHENOLS

✓ tannic acid

chlorogenic acid

phenolic acid

✓ oxalates

PER SERVING

IRON	heme iron	nonheme iron
	trace	4.5 mg

Squeeze the excess water out of the spinach by pressing with an absorbent paper towel. Set aside.

Cook the lasagna according to the package directions. Drain and rinse with cool water.

In a medium bowl mix the eggs, ricotta, and spinach together.

In a shallow glass casserole dish begin to layer the lasagna noodles, then spinach mixture, marinara sauce, mozzarella cheese, and Parmesan cheese. Continue to layer, ending with lasagna, reserving some marinara, mozzarella, and Parmesan. Spread a thin layer of marinara sauce over the noodles. Top with mozzarella and parmesan. Bake uncovered at 350° for 45 minutes to 1 hour.

Let stand 15 minutes before serving.

Serves 6

Stuffed Chicken Breasts

4   boneless, skinless chicken breasts
1   cup strong tea
1   cup garlic-seasoned croutons
1   3-ounce package Neufchâtel cheese
¼   cup Parmesan cheese
¼   teaspoon ground thyme
¼   teaspoon ground rosemary
¼   teaspoon ground basil
¼   teaspoon ground oregano
¼   cup buttermilk
¼   cup crisp crumbled bacon or bacon substitute

Rinse the chicken in cold water. Marinate overnight in tea.

Drain the chicken and pat dry. Place between sheets of waxed paper and pound with a meat mallet until flattened.

In a food processor grind up the croutons. In a medium bowl mix the cheeses, herbs, and crumbled bacon. Spread one-fourth of the mixture in the center of each piece of chicken and roll the chicken until closed. Dip in the buttermilk, then dredge in the seasoned crumbs. Place seam side down in a casserole dish. Cover and bake at 325° for 1 hour.

Serves 4

THIS RECIPE

is LOW in HEME iron and contains the following substances that inhibit absorption of nonheme iron:

calcium

dairy phosphate

eggs

phytate phosphorus

POLYPHENOLS

✓ tannic acid

chlorogenic acid

phenolic acid

✓ oxalates

PER SERVING

IRON	heme iron	nonheme iron
	0.4 mg	1.5 mg

Stuffed Shells with Three Fillings

CHEESE FILLING:

½	cup Ricotta cheese
½	cup shredded fontina cheese
½	cup shredded mozzarella cheese
1	egg
¼	teaspoon salt
¼	teaspoon white pepper

TOFU FILLING:

8	ounces tofu, drained
1	egg
¼	cup chopped green pepper
¼	cup chopped mushrooms
¼	cup finely chopped onion
2	tablespoons olive oil
1	teaspoon basil
1	teaspoon fresh parsley
¼	teaspoon salt
¼	teaspoon white pepper
1	teaspoon garlic powder

MEAT FILLING:

½	pound ground veal
¼	cup seedless rye bread crumbs
1	egg
¼	teaspoon salt
¼	teaspoon red pepper
1	teaspoon garlic powder
1	teaspoon basil
1	teaspoon fresh parsley

12	jumbo pasta shells
2	cups Marinara Sauce (see page 243)

In a medium bowl combine all of the ingredients for the desired filling.

Cook the pasta according to the package directions. Drain. Rinse with cold water, drain, and set aside.

Stuff each cooked pasta shell with 2 tablespoons of the filling. Pour a small amount of sauce in the bottom of a glass baking dish. Place the stuffed shells in the sauce and cover with the remaining sauce. Cover and bake at 350° for 40 minutes.

Uncover, turn off the oven, and let stand another 15 minutes in the oven.

Serves 6

THIS RECIPE

is LOW in HEME iron and contains the following substances that inhibit absorption of nonheme iron:

✓ calcium

✓ dairy phosphate

✓ eggs

✓ phytate phosphorus

POLYPHENOLS

✓ tannic acid

✓ chlorogenic acid

phenolic acid

✓ oxalates

PER SERVING

IRON	heme iron	nonheme iron
Cheese filling:	trace	0.78 mg
Tofu filling:	trace	0.9 mg
Meat filling:	trace	0.9 mg

The Hemochromatosis Cookbook

Stuffed Eggplant

1	medium eggplant
1	teaspoon salt
1/4	cup crumbled blue cheese
1/4	cup Parmesan cheese
1/4	cup bread crumbs
1	egg
1	tablespoon flour
1/2	teaspoon oregano
1/2	teaspoon basil
1/2	teaspoon thyme
1	6-ounce can tomato paste
3	cans hot coffee (2¼ cups)
1	teaspoon minced garlic
1/8	teaspoon black pepper
3/4	cup grated Swiss cheese

Preheat overn to 350°. Wash, dry, and split the eggplant lengthwise. Place in a shallow glass baking dish flesh side down. Add a small amount of water to the dish. Bake for 30 minutes.

Remove the eggplant. Scoop out the pulp and place in a mixing bowl. Add the remaining ingredients except the Swiss cheese. Pack the mixture into eggplant shells and top with the Swiss cheese. Bake uncovered at 350° for 40 minutes or until the top is golden brown.

Let stand 10 to 15 minutes before serving. Slice across the eggplant for each serving.

Serves 4

THIS RECIPE

is LOW in HEME iron and contains the following substances that inhibit absorption of nonheme iron:

calcium

✓ dairy phosphate

✓ eggs

phytate phosphorus

POLYPHENOLS

✓ tannic acid

chlorogenic acid

phenolic acid

✓ oxalates

PER SERVING

IRON	heme iron	nonheme iron
	0.4 mg	1.3 mg

Sweet-and-Sour Pork

½ cup oil
1 pound lean pork, trimmed and cut into thick strips
½ cup flour
¼ cup brewed strong coffee
1 cup broth
1 cup brewed strong black tea
½ teaspoon salt
1 cup wild rice
1 tablespoon olive oil
1 cup green pepper, cut in julienne strips
½ cup pineapple juice
1 cup soy sauce
½ cup brown sugar
1 tablespoon instant coffee
2 teaspoons cornstarch
¼ cup water

In a skillet heat the oil. Dredge the meat in flour and brown in the hot oil. Add the brewed coffee, cover, and reduce the heat. Continue slow cooking the meat for about 45 minutes.

Prepare the rice. In a stockpot bring the broth, tea, and salt to a boil. Add the rice. Cover, reduce the heat, and steam for 25 minutes.

When the meat is done, remove and set aside. Add 1 tablespoon of olive oil to the drippings and sauté the peppers for about 10 minutes. Remove the peppers and set aside along with the meat. Add the pineapple juice, soy sauce, brown sugar, and instant coffee to the meat drippings and bring to a boil.

In a shaker container mix the cornstarch and water. Shake vigorously and add to the boiling sauce with a whisk. Serve the thickened sauce over rice, add a serving of meat, and top with peppers.

Serves 6

This Recipe

is LOW in HEME iron and contains the following substances that inhibit absorption of nonheme iron:

✓ calcium
✓ dairy phosphate
eggs
✓ phytate phosphorus
POLYPHENOLS
✓ tannic acid
✓ chlorogenic acid
phenolic acid
oxalates

Per Serving

IRON	heme iron	nonheme iron
	0.7 mg	3.0 mg

The Hemochromatosis Cookbook

Tostidos

1	tablespoon olive oil
¼	cup finely chopped onion
1	tablespoon minced garlic
1	pound ground turkey
1	6-ounce can tomato paste
3	cans hot coffee (2¼ cups)
1	tablespoon cumin
1	teaspoon salt
2	tablespoons fresh chopped parsley
	Pinch red pepper
8	corn tortillas
1	cup Refried Beans (see page 68)
1½	cups shredded Monterey Jack cheese
4	cups shredded lettuce
1	cup avocado topping

In a saucepan heat the olive oil and sauté the onion and garlic. Add the meat and cook until the meat is done. Add the tomato paste, hot coffee, cumin, salt, parsley, and red pepper, and simmer until the mixture is thickened.

Preheat the oven to 350°. On each tortilla spread the refried beans. Add a layer of meat, and then cheese. Heat in the oven for 15 minutes. Remove and serve with shredded lettuce and avocado topping.

Serves 6 to 8

THIS RECIPE

is LOW in HEME iron and contains the following substances that inhibit absorption of nonheme iron:

✓ calcium

✓ dairy phosphate

eggs

✓ phytate phosphorus

POLYPHENOLS

✓ tannic acid

✓ chlorogenic acid

phenolic acid

oxalates

PER SERVING

IRON	heme iron	nonheme iron
	0.3 mg	2.5 mg

Tuna Casserole

2 quarts water
1 teaspoon salt
1 tablespoon instant tea
12 ounces whole-wheat noodles
1 cup Mushroom Velouté (see page 244)
½ cup reduced-fat sour cream
2 tablespoons mayonnaise
1 8-ounce can white water-packed tuna, drained
½ cup frozen peas
1 cup shredded Cheddar cheese

In a stockpot bring the water, salt, and tea bag to a boil. Drop the noodles into the boiling water, and cook according to the time specified on the package. Drain and rinse the noodles.

In a medium bowl combine the velouté, sour cream, and mayonnaise.

Spray an 8-inch square glass baking dish with vegetable spray. Layer noodles, a portion of sauce, all of the tuna, then the peas. Cover with the remaining sauce and the Cheddar cheese. Bake uncovered at 350° for 45 minutes.

6 servings

THIS RECIPE

is LOW in HEME iron and contains the following substances that inhibit absorption of nonheme iron:

✓ calcium

✓ dairy phosphate

eggs

✓ phytate phosphorus

POLYPHENOLS

✓ tannic acid

✓ chlorogenic acid

phenolic acid

oxalates

PER SERVING

IRON	heme iron	nonheme iron
	0.5 mg	2.4 mg

The Hemochromatosis Cookbook

Turkey Chili

1 tablespoon olive oil
½ cup finely chopped onion
1 pound fresh ground turkey
1 15¼-ounce can diced tomatoes
1 6-ounce can tomato paste
3 cans hot coffee (2¼ cups)
1 cup ketchup
1 teaspoon salt
½ teaspoon red pepper
1 15¼-ounce can dark red kidney
beans

In a saucepan heat the oil and sauté the onion. Add the meat and cook until done. Add the tomatoes and simmer for 15 minutes. Add the tomato paste, hot coffee, ketchup, and seasonings, and simmer for 30 minutes.

Rinse and drain the beans. Add to the chili and heat through.

Serves 4

THIS RECIPE

is LOW in HEME iron and contains the following substances that inhibit absorption of nonheme iron:

✓ calcium

✓ dairy phosphate

eggs

✓ phytate phosphorus

POLYPHENOLS

✓ tannic acid

✓ chlorogenic acid

phenolic acid

oxalates

PER SERVING

IRON	heme iron	nonheme iron
	0.6 mg	4.9 mg

Turkey Florentine Noodle Casserole

1	1¾-pound turkey breast
1	cup brewed strong black tea
2	parsnips, washed and trimmed
2	ribs celery with leaves
1	cup diced fresh tomatoes
1½	teaspoons salt
2	tablespoons coarse ground black pepper
7	cups water
1½	cups brewed strong black tea
10	ounces spinach noodles
4	cups strained turkey stock
¼	cup olive oil
¼	cup all-purpose flour
1	cup heavy cream
1	teaspoon salt
1	cup freshly grated Parmesan cheese
¼	teaspoon nutmeg

THIS RECIPE

*is LOW in HEME iron and contains
the following substances that
inhibit absorption of nonheme iron:*

✓ calcium

✓ dairy phosphate

eggs

✓ phytate phosphorus

POLYPHENOLS

✓ tannic acid

✓ chlorogenic acid

phenolic acid

oxalates

PER SERVING

IRON	heme iron	nonheme iron
	0.4 mg	2.2 mg

Preheat oven to 325°. Place the turkey breast, 1 cup of tea, parsnips, celery, tomatoes, ½ teaspoon of salt, and pepper in a cooking bag. Close the bag and bake for 2 hours.

In a stockpot bring the water to a boil with 1 teaspoon of salt and the tea added, and cook the spinach noodles until almost done. Drain, rinse, and set aside.

When the turkey is done, remove it from the oven bag and let cool for slicing. Place ½ cup of turkey stock plus the cooked vegetables in a food processor. Pulse and set aside.

In a saucepan heat the olive oil and whisk in the flour until a paste forms. Slowly add ½ cup of stock, then the puréed vegetables. As the mixture thickens, continue to pour in the stock until the sauce is the consistency of very thick gravy. Whisk in the cream and nutmeg. Heat through but do not boil. Season with 1 teaspoon of salt.

In a 9 x 13-inch glass casserole dish layer the noodles and sliced turkey, and cover with the sauce. Top with Parmesan. Bake uncovered at 400° for about 20 minutes.

Serves 8

The Hemochromatosis Cookbook

Leftover Thanksgiving Day Turkey Marsala

¼ cup olive oil, divided
¼ cup flour
1 cup brewed green tea
1 cup dry white wine
1 cup chicken broth
1 pound sliced mushrooms
¼ cup sour cream
1 pound cooked turkey, cut up
1 teaspoon salt
¼ teaspoon white pepper
2 cups cooked brown & wild rice blend

THIS RECIPE

is LOW in HEME iron and contains the following substances that inhibit absorption of nonheme iron:

calcium

dairy phosphate

eggs

phytate phosphorus

POLYPHENOLS

✓ tannic acid

chlorogenic acid

phenolic acid

oxalates

PER SERVING

IRON	heme iron	nonheme iron
	0.2 mg	0.3 mg

In a skillet over medium heat make a paste with half of the oil and the flour; stir with a whisk until brown.

Add green tea slowly to the flour mixture; while continuing to stir, add wine and broth slowly to maintain thick texture.

Meanwhile, in a separate skillet heat the remaining olive oil and sauté the mushrooms until tender.

Bring sauce to gentle boil; reduce temperature and stir in sour cream.

Add the turkey and the mushrooms. Season with salt ane pepper. Cook on low heat until meat is heated through. Spoon over hot wild rice.

Serves 4

Veal Moussaka

1   cup olive oil
1   eggplant
2   cups whole-wheat flour for dredging
2   eggs, lightly beaten
2   cups bread crumbs
2   tablespoons olive oil
¼   cup whole-wheat flour
1   teaspoon salt
¼   teaspoon white pepper
1   cup 1% milk
1   cup shredded Monterey Jack cheese
¼   cup grated Parmesan cheese
1   pound ground veal
2   cups Marinara Sauce (see page 243)
½   teaspoon cinnamon
½   teaspoon oregano
      Shredded Cheddar for topping
      Parmesan cheese for topping

THIS RECIPE

is LOW in HEME iron and contains the following substances that inhibit absorption of nonheme iron:

✓ calcium

✓ dairy phosphate

✓ eggs

✓ phytate phosphorus

POLYPHENOLS

✓ tannic acid

✓ chlorogenic acid

phenolic acid

oxalates

PER SERVING

IRON	heme iron	nonheme iron
	0.36 mg	2.2 mg

In a skillet heat 1 cup of olive oil over medium-high heat for frying.

Wash and dry the eggplant. Split the eggplant lengthwise, then again across into medium-width slices. In separate shallow dishes place 2 cups of whole-wheat flour, the eggs, and bread crumbs. Dredge the eggplant slices first in flour, then in the eggs, then in bread crumbs. Drop in hot olive oil, brown, turn and brown the other side.

Remove from the oil, and place on a paper towel to drain. Sprinkle salt lightly over the surface of the fried eggplant.

Prepare the cheese sauce. In a saucepan heat 2 tablespoons of olive oil. Whisk in ¼ cup of whole-wheat flour and add 1 teaspoon of salt and ¼ teaspoon of white pepper. Stir until light brown. Slowly add the milk, stirring until blended. Add the Monterey Jack and Parmesan cheeses, and heat until melted and smooth.

Prepare the meat sauce. In a skillet brown the veal. Drain and add the marinara sauce, cinnamon, and oregano.

Place the breaded eggplant in the bottom of a shallow glass casserole dish, overlapping each piece with the next. Cover with meat sauce, then cheese sauce. Top with shredded Cheddar and sprinkle with Parmesan. Bake uncovered at 350° for 45 minutes or until the top begins to brown.

Serves 6

Veal Stroganoff

1   **pound veal, cut into thick strips**
½   **cup hearty red wine (burgundy)**
½   **cup brewed black tea**
4   **tablespoons whole-wheat flour**
½   **cup olive oil**
½   **cup finely chopped onion**
1½   **cups sliced mushrooms**
1   **cup broth**
1   **cup sour cream**
     Cooked spinach noodles or wild rice

In a shallow dish marinate the meat overnight in the wine and tea.

Dredge the meat in flour. In a skillet heat the olive oil and sauté the meat until browned. Remove the meat and sauté the onion for 10 to 15 minutes. Add the mushrooms and sauté until tender. Return the meat to the skillet and add the broth and marinade. Simmer until the meat is tender and the liquid is reduced by half. Stir in the sour cream and heat through.

Serve over cooked spinach noodles or wild rice.

Serves 6

This Recipe

is LOW in HEME iron and contains the following substances that inhibit absorption of nonheme iron:

✓ calcium
✓ dairy phosphate
eggs
phytate phosphorus
POLYPHENOLS
✓ tannic acid
chlorogenic acid
phenolic acid
oxalates

Per Serving

IRON	heme iron	nonheme iron
	0.63 mg	1.96 mg

Veal Paprikash

¼   cup olive oil
1   pound veal, trimmed and cut into stew-size pieces
½   cup flour
½   cup finely chopped onion
1   tablespoon high-quality fresh ground paprika
½   cup chopped red bell pepper (green bell pepper if red is not available)
½   cup diced tomatoes
1   tablespoon tomato paste
1   cup brewed strong black tea
1   cup sour cream
    Tiny Dumplings (recipe below)

TINY DUMPLINGS:
1   cup flour
½   teaspoon salt
½   cup brewed black tea
2   quarts water

In a skillet heat the oil. Dredge the meat in flour and brown in the hot oil. Set the meat aside. Add the onion and sauté until tender. Add the paprika, pepper, tomatoes, paste, and tea. Bring to a gentle boil to thicken. Return the meat to the sauce and heat through. Stir in the sour cream. Serve over Tiny Dumplings.

Sift together the flour and salt. Add the tea, and mix until a dough forms. Place the dough on a floured pastry cloth and roll out until about ¼ inch thick. Cut into ½-inch-wide strips, and cut each strip into ½-inch dumplings. Drop into boiling water. Dumplings will float when done. Scoop out and set aside.

Serves 6

THIS RECIPE

is LOW in HEME iron and contains the following substances that inhibit absorption of nonheme iron:

✓ calcium

✓ dairy phosphate

eggs

✓ phytate phosphorus

POLYPHENOLS

✓ tannic acid

✓ chlorogenic acid

phenolic acid

oxalates

PER SERVING

IRON	heme iron	nonheme iron
	0.7 mg	2.3 mg

Webb's "Faux Bacon"

2   ounces very lean ham, thinly
    sliced
1   cup olive oil

Bacon does not contain much iron but it is high in fat. It offers great flavor to recipes and should not necessarily be eliminated from one's diet unless instructed to do so by a physician. One alternative to regular bacon is Webb's "faux bacon."

While owning and operating a very busy family restaurant, sometimes the owners would find the kitchen out of something needed. With no time to go to the store, Webb Garrison, husband of author Cheryl Garrison, often devised creative substitutes. During one such event when the kitchen ran out of bacon and several orders for club sandwiches needed to be filled, "faux bacon" was invented. Webb grabbed a slab of deli ham, sliced several pieces on the meat slicer, then cut each piece into long strips similar to the shape of bacon. He then dropped the pieces into hot oil. Customers reported they enjoyed their club sandwiches and that the "bacon" was delicious.

Because olive oil is used as its fat, "faux bacon" is a bit healthier than regular bacon, though it contains about the same amount of sodium.

For the best type of ham, look in the lunch meat section for reduced sodium/fat ham.

Cut the ham lengthwise into $1/2$-inch-wide slices.

Method #1: Pour the olive oil into a shallow glass cooking dish. Place in a 425° oven until the oil is heated. Place strips of ham in the oil and return to the oven. Ham will fry just like regular bacon with sufficient oil and heat. For best results, be certain to get the oil very hot before adding the ham.

Method #2: In a skillet heat the olive oil. Place strips of ham in the hot oil. Ham will fry just like regular bacon with sufficient oil and heat.

PER SERVING

IRON	heme iron	nonheme iron
	trace	trace

Vegetable Lasagna

2	cups chopped broccoli
1	tablespoon water
2	tablespoons olive oil
1	cup finely chopped onion
1	tablespoon minced garlic
1	cup sliced mushrooms
1	cup chopped green pepper
½	teaspoon salt
7	cups water
1	cup brewed strong black tea
1	teaspoon salt
9	medium width lasagna noodles
1	cup ricotta cheese
2	eggs
¼	cup fresh chopped parsley
½	teaspoon dried thyme, crushed
½	teaspoon dried marjoram, crushed
2	tablespoons capers
½	cup black olives
¼	teaspoon red pepper
1	cup shredded mozzarella cheese
4	cups Marinara Sauce (see page 243)
½	cup grated Parmesan cheese

Chop the broccoli into very small pieces. Place in a microwave safe glass bowl with 1 tablespoon of water. Cover with plastic wrap and cook on medium-high for 2 minutes or until tender.

In a skillet heat 2 tablespoons of oil and sauté the onion and minced garlic until tender, about 15 minutes. Add the mushrooms and cook until tender and no liquid remains.

Add the green pepper, and continue cooking about 5 to 7 minutes until the peppers are tender. Sprinkle the cooked vegetables with ½ teaspoon of salt.

(continued on next page)

THIS RECIPE

is LOW in HEME iron and contains the following substances that inhibit absorption of nonheme iron:

✓ calcium

✓ dairy phosphate

✓ eggs

✓ phytate phosphorus

POLYPHENOLS

✓ tannic acid

✓ chlorogenic acid

phenolic acid

✓ oxalates

PER SERVING

IRON	heme iron	nonheme iron
	trace	1.56 mg

In a stockpot bring the water, tea, and 1 teaspoon of salt to a boil. Drop the lasagna noodles into the boiling tea-water and cook until tender, about 10 minutes. Drain and rinse.

Mix together the ricotta cheese, egg, herbs, capers, olives, and red pepper.

Spray the bottom of a 9 x 13-inch glass baking dish with vegetable spray. Place 3 noodles lengthwise in the dish. Begin layers of cheese mixture, mushroom-onion mixture, then broccoli, and mozzarella. Spoon about $^2/_3$ cup of marinara sauce over the layers and top with Parmesan cheese. Repeat with another layer in the same sequence, ending with a layer of noodles topped with sauce and Parmesan. Reserve additional sauce for individual servings.

Cover and bake at 375° for 30 minutes.

Uncover and bake an additional 10 minutes. Let stand for 10 to 15 minutes before serving.

Serves 8

Asparagus with Lemon Caraway Sauce

3/4   **pound fresh asparagus**
1   **cup tea**
1   **ounce fresh lemon juice**
1/2   **teaspoon caraway seed**
1   **tablespoon cornstarch**
1/4   **cup sour cream**
1/2   **teaspoon salt**
   Pinch white pepper

THIS RECIPE

is LOW in HEME iron and contains the following substances that inhibit absorption of nonheme iron:

✓ calcium

✓ dairy phosphate

✓ eggs

✓ phytate phosphorus

POLYPHENOLS

✓ tannic acid

✓ chlorogenic acid

phenolic acid

✓ oxalates

PER SERVING

IRON	heme iron	nonheme iron
	trace	1.56 mg

Wash the asparagus and snap off the woody ends. In a saucepan bring the tea to a boil with the lemon juice. Add the asparagus and caraway and simmer in the liquid until tender. Remove the asparagus and bring the liquid to a boil. In a shaker mix the cornstarch with a bit of water and shake to mix well. Add the cornstarch mixture to the cooking liquid and whisk constantly until thick. Add the sour cream. Season with salt and pepper.

Serves 4

Artichoke Asparagus Casserole

1   egg, lightly beaten
1/2   cup egg substitute
1   3-ounce package Neufchâtel cheese
1/4   cup shredded Parmesan cheese
3/4   teaspoon garlic powder
1/4   teaspoon white pepper
1/4   cup strong brewed tea
1/2   cup Pepperidge Farm® stuffing mix
3/4   cup shredded Swiss cheese
1   cup ricotta cheese
3/4   cup shredded Vermont or New York sharp Cheddar cheese
1   small jar artichoke hearts
1   cup chopped frozen asparagus
1   tablespoon fresh chopped parsley
1   tablespoon oregano
1   2-ounce jar diced pimientos, drained

In a large bowl mix the egg, egg substitute, Neufchâtel cheese, Parmesan cheese, garlic powder, and pepper. Add the tea, stuffing mix, Swiss, ricotta, and half the Cheddar cheese. Dice the artichoke hearts and add to the mixture along with the asparagus, parsley, oregano, and pimientos.

Spray a glass casserole dish with vegetable spray and place the mixture in the dish. Bake at 350° for about 30 minutes.

Top with the remaining Cheddar cheese and bake for an additional 10 to 15 minutes. Let stand for 10 minutes before serving.

Serves 4 to 6

THIS RECIPE

is LOW in HEME iron and contains the following substances that inhibit absorption of nonheme iron:

✓ calcium

✓ dairy phosphate

✓ eggs

✓ phytate phosphorus

POLYPHENOLS

✓ tannic acid

✓ chlorogenic acid

phenolic aci

oxalates

PER SERVING

IRON	heme iron	nonheme iron
	trace	1.97 mg

     The Hemochromatosis Cookbook

Baked Beans

⅓ cup brown sugar
½ cup strong coffee
¼ cup vinegar
1 cup ketchup
1 teaspoon dry mustard
1 28-ounce can pork and beans, drained
½ cup chopped onion

In a saucepan combine the brown sugar, coffee, vinegar, ketchup, and dry mustard, and simmer for 5 to 10 minutes.

In a casserole dish layer the beans, onions, and sauce mixture. Cover and bake at 350° for 40 minutes.

Uncover and bake at 400° for 20 minutes.

Remove from the oven and let stand 10 minutes before serving.

Serves 4

THIS RECIPE

is LOW in HEME iron and contains the following substances that inhibit absorption of nonheme iron:

✓ calcium

✓ dairy phosphate

eggs

✓ phytate phosphorus

POLYPHENOLS

✓ tannic acid

✓ chlorogenic acid

phenolic acid

oxalates

PER SERVING

IRON	heme iron	nonheme iron
	0.0 mg	2.5 mg

Baked Beets with Apple Glaze

1   **bunch fresh beets**
1   **cup apple juice**
1   **teaspoon cornstarch**

THIS RECIPE

*is LOW in HEME iron and contains
the following substances that
inhibit absorption of nonheme iron:*

calcium

dairy phosphate

eggs

✓ phytate phosphorus

POLYPHENOLS

tannic acid

chlorogenic acid

✓ phenolic acid

oxalates

PER SERVING

IRON	heme iron	nonheme iron
	0.0 mg	0.7 mg

Rinse the beets well and cut off the stems and roots.

Preheat the oven to 350°. Place the beets in a glass cooking dish and bake uncovered for about 1 hour; a fork or knife will slide in easily when the beet is done.

In a saucepan bring the apple juice to a boil. In a shaker mix the cornstarch with a bit of water and shake to mix well. Add the cornstarch mixture to the apple juice and whisk constantly until thick. Remove the beets from the oven and top with the apple glaze.

Serves 4

Baked Rice

¼   cup olive oil
¼   cup finely chopped onion
1   teaspoon minced garlic
½   cup chopped fresh tomatoes
2   cups chicken broth
1   cup brewed tea
1   teaspoon salt
     Pinch red pepper
1½   cups uncooked basmati rice
½   cup finely chopped spinach
¼   cup chopped fresh parsley
2   sprigs thyme or ½ teaspoon dried thyme
1   bay leaf

Preheat the oven to 425°. In a skillet heat the oil and sauté the onion and garlic until golden. Add the tomatoes and cook until tender.

Add the broth, tea, salt, pepper, rice, spinach, parsley, thyme, and bay leaf. Cover and bake for 40 minutes.

Turn off the oven and let stand without opening the oven door for 20 to 30 minutes.

Remove the bay leaf before serving.

Serves 6 to 8

THIS RECIPE

is LOW in HEME iron and contains the following substances that inhibit absorption of nonheme iron:

calcium
✓ dairy phosphate
eggs
✓ phytate phosphorus
POLYPHENOLS
✓ tannic acid
✓ chlorogenic acid
phenolic acid
✓ oxalates

PER SERVING

IRON	heme iron	nonheme iron
	0.0 mg	2.1 mg

Broccoli Casserole

1   10-ounce box chopped broccoli, thawed but not cooked (leftover broccoli works fine also)

1   cup cooked rice (prepared in broth-tea mixture or use leftover baked rice)

$\frac{1}{2}$ cup cottage cheese

1   cup Hollandaise sauce (Knorr Swiss brand, 1 package prepared)

1   cup shredded sharp Cheddar cheese

1   egg

1   tablespoon flour

1   teaspoon salt

$\frac{1}{2}$ teaspoon white pepper

Preheat the oven to 350°. In a large bowl combine all of the ingredients. Lightly oil a glass baking dish and pour the mixture into the dish. Bake uncovered for 45 minutes.

Let stand 10 minutes before serving.

Serves 4

THIS RECIPE

is LOW in HEME iron and contains the following substances that inhibit absorption of nonheme iron:

✓ calcium

✓ dairy phosphate

✓ eggs

✓ phytate phosphorus

POLYPHENOLS

✓ tannic acid

✓ chlorogenic acid

phenolic acid

✓ oxalates

PER SERVING

IRON	heme iron	nonheme iron
	0.0 mg	2.8 mg

Brussels Sprouts with Sour Cream and Dill

2	cups fresh Brussels sprouts
1/4	cup olive oil
1	cup sour cream
	Pinch black pepper
1	teaspoon dill weed

Wash the sprouts and cut off the stems. Cut the sprouts in half. In a skillet heat olive oil over medium-high heat. When oil is hot, place sprouts flat-side down. Cook until sprouts are golden dark brown and tender when pierced with a fork.

In a saucepan heat the sour cream and pepper, and add the dill. Serve over the Brussels sprouts.

Serves 4

THIS RECIPE

is LOW in HEME iron and contains the following substances that inhibit absorption of nonheme iron:

✓ calcium

✓ dairy phosphate

eggs

✓ phytate phosphorus

POLYPHENOLS

✓ tannic acid

✓ chlorogenic acid

phenolic acid

oxalates

PER SERVING

IRON	heme iron	nonheme iron
	0.0 mg	0.5 mg

Cabbage and Onions
with Black Pepper

½ cup olive oil
½ yellow onion finely, chopped
½ head green cabbage, chopped
½ teaspoon salt
    Black pepper
½ cup brewed tea

In a skillet heat the oil and sauté the onion until tender. Increase the heat and add the cabbage. Stir so the onion is mixed with the cabbage. Add salt to taste and generous amounts of black pepper. Add the tea, cover, and steam for 30 minutes.

Serves 4

THIS RECIPE

is LOW in HEME iron and contains the following substances that inhibit absorption of nonheme iron:

calcium

✓ dairy phosphate

eggs

✓ phytate phosphorus

POLYPHENOLS

✓ tannic acid

✓ chlorogenic acid

phenolic acid

oxalates

PER SERVING

IRON	heme iron	nonheme iron
	0.0 mg	0.3 mg

Cabbage Casserole

2 tablespoons olive oil
½ cup finely chopped onion
½ head green cabbage, chopped
1 cup brewed tea
½ teaspoon salt
½ teaspoon black pepper
¼ teaspoon caraway seeds
1 egg
½ cup light cream
⅔ cup seasoned bread stuffing
⅔ cup shredded Swiss cheese
¼ cup Parmesan cheese

Preheat oven to 350°. In a stockpot heat the olive oil and sauté the onion until tender. Add the cabbage and tea, and cook the until the cabbage is tender. Add salt, pepper, and caraway seeds.

In a medium bowl combine the egg and cream. In an oiled glass 8-inch square baking dish layer the cabbage onion mixture, then stuffing, then Swiss cheese, reserving a small amount to put on top. Pour the cream mixture over the top. Sprinkle with the remaining Swiss and Parmesan cheeses. Bake uncovered for about 40 minutes.

Serves 4

THIS RECIPE

is LOW in HEME iron and contains the following substances that inhibit absorption of nonheme iron:

✓ calcium

✓ dairy phosphate

✓ eggs

✓ phytate phosphorus

POLYPHENOLS

✓ tannic acid

✓ chlorogenic acid

phenolic acid

oxalates

PER SERVING

IRON	heme iron	nonheme iron
	0.0 mg	0.5 mg

Confetti Vegetable Casserole

1 tablespoon olive oil
½ cup finely chopped onion
2 tablespoons minced garlic
1 cup sliced fresh mushrooms
½ cup brown rice
½ cup wild rice
1 teaspoon salt
½ teaspoon white pepper
1½ cups turkey or chicken broth
½ cup brewed tea
¼ cup shredded carrot
¼ cup chopped fresh spinach
½ cup frozen asparagus pieces (thawed but not cooked)
½ cup diced tomato
2 tablespoons fresh chopped parsley
1 egg, lightly beaten
2 tablespoons whole-wheat flour
1 cup cubed havarti cheese
¼ cup grated Parmesan cheese
2 cups Mushroom Velouté (see page 244)

In a skillet heat the olive oil and sauté the onion and garlic until tender. Add the mushrooms and cook until tender. Add the rices, salt, white pepper, broth, and tea, and bring to a boil. Cover, reduce the heat, and allow the rice to steam for 25 minutes (brown rice may take longer).

Preheat oven to 350°. In a large mixing bowl combine the vegetables, parsley, egg, and flour. Add the rice, cheeses, and velouté.

Spray a casserole dish with vegetable spray. Pack the ingredients into the casserole dish. Bake uncovered at 350° for 45 minutes or until the center puffs up and begins to brown.

Serves 4 to 6

THIS RECIPE

is LOW in HEME iron and contains the following substances that inhibit absorption of nonheme iron:

✓ calcium

✓ dairy phosphate

✓ eggs

✓ phytate phosphorus

POLYPHENOLS

✓ tannic acid

✓ chlorogenic acid

phenolic acid

oxalates

PER SERVING

IRON	heme iron	nonheme iron
	0.0 mg	0.5 mg

Dressing (Stuffing)

¼ cup olive oil
½ cup finely chopped onion
½ cup chopped celery
6 cups whole-wheat bread cubes
4 cups leftover corn bread (tear apart and let stand in open air overnight)
2 tablespoons chopped fresh parsley
3 cups turkey or chicken broth
1 cup brewed tea
2 tablespoons salt
4 tablespoons rubbed sage
1 teaspoon black pepper
2 eggs, lightly beaten

In a skillet heat the oil and sauté the onion and celery until tender. In a large bowl stir all of the ingredients together, adding the eggs last. Pack into a glass baking dish. Bake uncovered at 375° for 45 minutes.

Let stand 10 minutes before serving.

Serves 10 to 12

THIS RECIPE

is LOW in HEME iron and contains the following substances that inhibit absorption of nonheme iron:

calcium

✓ dairy phosphate

✓ eggs

✓ phytate phosphorus

POLYPHENOLS

✓ tannic acid

✓ chlorogenic acid

phenolic acid

✓ oxalates

PER SERVING

IRON	heme iron	nonheme iron
	0.2 mg	3.15 mg

Dried Beans

8 cups broth

2 cups brewed tea

1 pound dried beans (navy, pinto, black, lima, or any personal favorite)

1 teaspoon salt

1 tablespoon olive oil

THIS RECIPE

is LOW in HEME iron and contains the following substances that inhibit absorption of nonheme iron:

calcium

✓ dairy phosphate

eggs

✓ phytate phosphorus

POLYPHENOLS

✓ tannic acid

✓ chlorogenic acid

phenolic acid

oxalates

PER SERVING

IRON	heme iron	nonheme iron
	0.0 mg	2.4 mg

In a stockpot bring to a boil the broth, oil, tea, and beans.

Add the salt and continue cooking the beans until tender, about 2 hours.

Serves 4 to 6

The Hemochromatosis Cookbook

Funny Fries

1   dozen new (red) potatoes
¼   cup olive oil
     Salt to taste

According to the National Cancer Institute, in the United States between the years 1970 and 1994, per-person consumption of vegetables increased by 19 percent. The potato topped the list of favorite vegetables. Unfortunately more than 50 percent of potatoes eaten are consumed as French fries, which joins the ranks of soft drinks, candy and refined sugar as unhealthy foods Americans consume in excess.

Potatoes are rich in fiber, with a whopping 4 grams per cup when eaten with the skins. They also contain calcium, magnesium, potassium, and folate. Prepared with olive oil, which is high in monounsaturated fat—the good kind of fat—potatoes with skins offer a healthy alternative to deep-fat-fried potatoes.

Wash and cut the potatoes in half; place in cold water to preserve. Oil the bottom of a large shallow glass baking dish. Shake salt onto the oil.

Preheat the oven to 450°. Place the dish in the oven to heat the oil (about 5 to 7 minutes once the oven is at temperature). Dry the potatoes with paper towels. Remove the dish from the oven. Place the potatoes face down in the hot oil. Return to the oven and bake for 15 to 20 minutes. The meat side of the potato should be golden brown, not black. Cut off the oven and let the potatoes stand in the oven for about 20 minutes.

THIS RECIPE

is LOW in HEME iron and contains the following substances that inhibit absorption of nonheme iron:

calcium

dairy phosphate

eggs

✓ phytate phosphorus

POLYPHENOLS

tannic acid

chlorogenic acid

phenolic acid

oxalates

PER SERVING

IRON	heme iron	nonheme iron
	trace	2.1 mg

Herbed Olive Oil
with Crusty French Bread

1 loaf French bread
$\frac{1}{2}$ cup extra virgin olive oil
1 tablespoon spicy mustard
1 tablespoon fresh parsley
$\frac{1}{4}$ teaspoon fresh cracked pepper

Bake the bread uncovered at 375° until crusty and brown, about 10 to 15 minutes. In a small bowl combine the olive oil, mustard, parsley, and pepper. Place the crusty hot bread and olive oil for dipping on the dinner table. Tear off pieces of bread and dip in olive oil.

Serves 4

THIS RECIPE

is LOW in HEME iron and contains the following substances that inhibit absorption of nonheme iron:

calcium

dairy phosphate

eggs

✓ phytate phosphorus

POLYPHENOLS

tannic acid

chlorogenic acid

phenolic acid

oxalates

PER SERVING

IRON	heme iron	nonheme iron
	0.0 mg	0.6 mg

Italian Green Bean Casserole

2   14.5-ounce cans Italian cut green beans, drained

⅓   teaspoon oregano

⅓   cup Parmesan cheese

½   cup light cream

1   cup Mushroom Velouté (see page 244)

1   cup Pepperidge Farm® bread stuffing mix

In a medium bowl mix the beans, oregano, Parmesan, cream, and velouté.

Spray a glass casserole dish with vegetable spray. Distribute half the stuffing mix over the bottom. Pour the beans and sauce over the stuffing mix. Top with the remaining stuffing mix. Bake at 400° for 40 minutes.

Serves 8

THIS RECIPE

is LOW in HEME iron and contains the following substances that inhibit absorption of nonheme iron:

✓ calcium

✓ dairy phosphate

eggs

✓ phytate phosphorus

POLYPHENOLS

✓ tannic acid

✓ chlorogenic acid

phenolic acid

oxalates

PER SERVING

IRON	heme iron	nonheme iron
	trace	0.8 mg

Kohlrabi Alfredo with Cracked Pepper

2   to 3 kohlrabi bulbs
1   cup brewed tea
1   cup Alfredo sauce
1   teaspoon coarse ground or fresh
     cracked black pepper

In a steamer place the kohlrabi bulbs and steam in the tea until tender. Cut the bulbs in half and spoon the Alfredo sauce over the kohlrabi. Sprinkle generously with fresh ground black pepper.

Serves 4

THIS RECIPE

is LOW in HEME iron and contains the following substances that inhibit absorption of nonheme iron:

✓ calcium

✓ dairy phosphate

eggs

✓ phytate phosphorus

POLYPHENOLS

✓ tannic acid

✓ chlorogenic acid

phenolic acid

oxalates

PER SERVING

IRON	heme iron	nonheme iron
	0.0 mg	0.3 mg

Kasha and Bowties with Chopped Kale

6	ounces bowtie pasta
7	cups water
1	teaspoon instant tea
1	teaspoon salt
2	tablespoons olive oil
1	cup finely chopped onion
1	teaspoon minced garlic
1	cup sliced mushrooms
1	cup chopped kale
1	teaspoon salt and black pepper
1	egg
1	cup kasha
2	cups hot chicken broth
1	teaspoon instant tea

In a stockpot cook the pasta in salted boiling water and the tea for about 8 minutes or until al dente. Drain, rinse, and set aside.

In a skillet heat the olive oil and sauté the onion and garlic for 15 minutes. Add the mushrooms and sauté until the liquid evaporates. Add the kale and season with salt and pepper. Cover and cook until the kale is done.

In a mixing bowl beat the egg and stir in the kasha, mixing until all kernels are coated.

In a glass skillet on medium-high heat cook the kasha, stirring constantly until the grains are toasted. Add the hot broth and tea, and simmer for about 8 minutes. Do not overcook or the kasha will become mushy. Add the pasta and the kale mixture, and mix well.

Serves 8

THIS RECIPE

is LOW in HEME iron and contains the following substances that inhibit absorption of nonheme iron:

✓ calcium

✓ dairy phosphate

eggs

✓ phytate phosphorus

POLYPHENOLS

✓ tannic acid

✓ chlorogenic acid

phenolic acid

✓ oxalates

PER SERVING

IRON	heme iron	nonheme iron
	trace	1.2 mg

Lima Bean Casserole

½ pound dry baby limas
7 cups water plus 1 cup brewed tea
1 teaspoon salt
2 strips bacon
1 tablespoon olive oil
¼ cup finely chopped onion
½ cup sour cream
1 cup Mushroom Velouté (see page 244)
¼ cup Parmesan cheese

In a stockpot simmer the limas in the water and tea seasoned with salt until tender.

Microwave the bacon strips until very crisp, drain, and set aside.

In a skillet heat the olive oil and sauté the onion until translucent. In a small bowl mix the sour cream and mushroom velouté, and add to the onion. Spray a square glass baking dish with vegetable spray. In the bottom of the dish layer limas, then sauce. Top with Parmesan and crumbled bacon. Bake uncovered at 350° for 45 minutes.

Serves 6 to 8

THIS RECIPE

is LOW in HEME iron and contains the following substances that inhibit absorption of nonheme iron:

✓ calcium

✓ dairy phosphate

eggs

✓ phytate phosphorus

POLYPHENOLS

✓ tannic acid

✓ chlorogenic acid

phenolic acid

oxalates

PER SERVING

IRON	heme iron	nonheme iron
	trace	3.2 mg

Macaroni and Cheese

1 16-ounce box whole-wheat elbow noodles
7 cups water
1 cup brewed tea
1 teaspoon salt
1 tablespoon olive oil
2 tablespoons oat bran blend flour
1 cup lowfat milk
½ cup diced Velveeta cheese
½ cup shredded sharp Cheddar

THIS RECIPE

is LOW in HEME iron and contains the following substances that inhibit absorption of nonheme iron:

✓ calcium

✓ dairy phosphate

eggs

✓ phytate phosphorus

POLYPHENOLS

✓ tannic acid

✓ chlorogenic acid

phenolic acid

oxalates

PER SERVING

IRON	heme iron	nonheme iron
	trace	3.2 mg

In a large pot cook the elbow noodles in the water and tea with salt until tender.

In the top of a double boiler over simmering water heat the olive oil. Add the oat bran flour and beat with a whisk until blended. Add the milk and continue to beat with a whisk until thickened. Add the Velveeta and Cheddar and gently mix. Whisk vigorously, scraping bottom edges gently with a wooden spoon. Pour the cheese sauce over cooked and rinsed macaroni. Cover and bake at 350° for 40 minutes.

Drink tea or coffee with this meal.

Serves 8

Okra with Lime Sauce

1   pound okra
½   cup brewed tea
½   teaspoon salt
2   tablespoons milk
3   ounces Neufchâtel cheese, cut into cubes
1   ounce fresh lime juice

Wash the okra and cut off the stems. Steam in tea and salt.

In a separate pan heat the milk. Add the cheese and warm until melted. Add the lime juice and whisk until blended. Top steamed okra with the lime sauce.

Serves 6

THIS RECIPE

is LOW in HEME iron and contains the following substances that inhibit absorption of nonheme iron:

✓ calcium

✓ dairy phosphate

eggs

✓ phytate phosphorus

POLYPHENOLS

✓ tannic acid

✓ chlorogenic acid

phenolic acid

✓ oxalates

PER SERVING

IRON	heme iron	nonheme iron
	0.0 mg	0.4 mg

Pasta

1   cup flour
1   teaspoon salt
1   egg
7   cups broth
1   cup brewed tea
¼   teaspoon salt

THIS RECIPE

*is LOW in HEME iron and contains
the following substances that
inhibit absorption of nonheme iron:*

calcium
✓ dairy phosphate
✓ eggs
✓ phytate phosphorus
POLYPHENOLS
✓ tannic acid
✓ chlorogenic acid
phenolic acid
oxalates

PER SERVING

IRON	heme iron	nonheme iron
	0.2 mg	0.5 mg

In a medium bowl combine the flour and salt. Place the flour mixture on a pastry cloth and create a well in the center. Break the egg into the well and blend the flour into the egg. Knead slightly, but do not overmix. Press the pasta down and sprinkle with flour. Dust the rolling pin with flour and roll out the pasta into thin sheets (get the sheets as thin as possible). Let dry for 2 hours.

Cut into 4-inch-wide strips. If the centers are still damp allow the pasta to dry another hour.

Stack the strips and beginning at one end cut ¼-inch-wide noodles. Toss with flour and drop into boiling broth with tea and salt. Simmer until tender, about 20 minutes.

Serves 4

Red Beans and Rice

7   cups water
     Ham bone with ½ cup ham
     pieces
1   pound red beans
2   cups brewed tea
1   teaspoon salt
1½   cups broth
½   cup brewed tea
1   teaspoon salt
1   teaspoon olive oil
1   cup rice
     Chopped spring onions

In a large pot bring the water to a boil. Add the ham bone, ham, beans, and 2 cups of tea. Reduce the heat and simmer the beans for 1 hour.

Add the salt and continue cooking the beans until tender.

In a separate pot bring the broth and ½ cup of tea to boil and add the salt, oil, and rice. Cover and steam for 25 minutes.

Spoon the beans over the rice. Top with chopped spring onions and serve with corn bread.

Serves 4 to 6

THIS RECIPE

is LOW in HEME iron and contains the following substances that inhibit absorption of nonheme iron:

calcium

✓ dairy phosphate

eggs

✓ phytate phosphorus

POLYPHENOLS

✓ tannic acid

✓ chlorogenic acid

phenolic acid

oxalates

PER SERVING

IRON	heme iron	nonheme iron
	0.2 mg	4.5 mg

Oven-Roasted Red Potatoes with Rosemary

12	red potatoes
	Olive oil
	Salt and pepper
2	tablespoons butter, melted
3	tablespoons olive oil
1	cup sour cream
2	tablespoons fresh rosemary
2	tablespoons chives
	Salt and pepper

THIS RECIPE

*is LOW in HEME iron and contains
the following substances that
inhibit absorption of nonheme iron:*

✓ calcium

✓ dairy phosphate

eggs

✓ phytate phosphorus

POLYPHENOLS

tannic acid

chlorogenic acid

phenolic acid

oxalates

PER SERVING

IRON	heme iron	nonheme iron
	0.0 mg	2.3 mg

Preheat the oven to 400°. Wash and cut the potatoes into halves. Coat a cookie sheet with olive oil, and lightly sprinkle with salt and pepper.

Place the cookie sheet in the oven for about 5 minutes until hot. Place the red potatoes cut side down on the hot sheet. Bake for 20 to 25 minutes until the potatoes are done (pierce with a fork).

While the potatoes are baking, prepare the sauce. In a small saucepan over low heat combine the butter, oil, and sour cream. Add the rosemary and chives. Pour the sauce over the roasted potatoes. Season with salt and pepper to taste.

Potatoes prepared this way are a great substitute for French fries.

Drink tea or coffee with this meal.

Serves 4 to 6

Shiitaki Mushrooms
with Feta Cheese and Herbs

1   tablespoon olive oil
12   cleaned shiitaki mushrooms
1   teaspoon rosemary
1   teaspoon fresh chopped parsley
1   teaspoon chopped chives
     Pinch red pepper
½   cup feta cheese

Brush olive oil on the mushrooms and sprinkle with herbs. Place under the broiler for 5 to 7 minutes. Remove and sprinkle with red pepper and feta cheese.

Serves 4

THIS RECIPE

is LOW in HEME iron and contains the following substances that inhibit absorption of nonheme iron:

✓ calcium

✓ dairy phosphate

eggs

✓ phytate phosphorus

POLYPHENOLS

✓ tannic acid

chlorogenic acid

phenolic acid

✓ oxalates

PER SERVING

IRON	heme iron	nonheme iron
	0.0 mg	0.4 mg

Shoepeg Corn with Roasted Red Peppers and Neufchâtel

¼ red bell pepper
1 tablespoon olive oil
1 10-ounce package frozen white shoepeg corn
½ cup brewed tea
3 ounces Neufchâtel cheese

Wash and seed the red pepper quarter. Brush the pepper quarter with olive oil and cut into thin strips. Place under the broiler until roasted (3 to 4 minutes; the pepper will be charred). Allow to cool.

In a steamer pot steam the corn in the tea. Chop the Neufchâtel and drop it into the corn. Chop the red pepper and add to the corn. Heat until the cheese melts.

Serves 6

THIS RECIPE

is LOW in HEME iron and contains the following substances that inhibit absorption of nonheme iron:

✓ calcium

✓ dairy phosphate

eggs

✓ phytate phosphorus

POLYPHENOLS

✓ tannic acid

✓ chlorogenic acid

phenolic acid

oxalates

PER SERVING

IRON	heme iron	nonheme iron
	0.0 mg	0.6 mg

Spinach Casserole

2 tablespoons olive oil
½ cup minced onion
2 eggs
½ cup lowfat milk
2 tablespoons chopped parsley
½ teaspoon salt
¼ teaspoon white pepper
½ cup cream cheese
1½ pounds fresh spinach
1½ cups rice
1 cup Swiss cheese (reserve ¼ cup for topping)
4 strips bacon, cooked and crumbled

In a skillet heat the oil and sauté the onion. In a medium bowl beat the eggs. Add the milk, onion, parsley, salt, and pepper. Add the cream cheese, spinach, rice, and ¾ cup of Swiss cheese, and pour into a greased shallow baking dish. Top with the remaining cheese and bacon. Bake uncovered at 350° for 40 to 45 minutes.

Let stand before serving.

Serves 6

This Recipe

is LOW in HEME iron and contains the following substances that inhibit absorption of nonheme iron:

✓ calcium

✓ dairy phosphate

eggs

phytate phosphorus

POLYPHENOLS

tannic acid

chlorogenic acid

phenolic acid

✓ oxalates

Per Serving

IRON	heme iron	nonheme iron
	trace	0.9 mg

Squash Casserole

3	pounds yellow squash
4	tablespoons olive oil
1	medium onion, coarsely chopped
1	teaspoon salt
1/4	teaspoon white pepper
1	cup brewed tea
2	cups Mushroom Velouté (see page 244) or 1 small can cream of mushroom soup
1	cup reduced-fat sour cream
1½	cups extra-sharp Cheddar cheese (Vermont or New York)
2	cups Pepperidge Farm® stuffing mix

Preheat the oven to 350°. Rinse the squash, remove the stems, cut up, and set aside.

In a skillet heat the oil and sauté the onion until tender. Add the squash, salt, pepper and tea, and simmer until tender.

Lightly oil a baking dish with olive oil or vegetable spray.

In a medium bowl mix the mushroom velouté and sour cream.

In the prepared baking dish alternate layers of squash-onion mixture, then sauce, Cheddar cheese, and Pepperidge Farm brand stuffing mix. Continue layering, ending with stuffing mix as topping. Bake uncovered for 45 minutes.

Serves 8 to 10

This Recipe

is LOW in HEME iron and contains the following substances that inhibit absorption of nonheme iron:

✓ calcium

✓ dairy phosphate

eggs

phytate phosphorus

POLYPHENOLS

✓ tannic acid

chlorogenic acid

phenolic acid

oxalates

Per Serving

IRON	heme iron	nonheme iron
	0.4 mg	0.24 mg

Twice-Baked Potato

4   Idaho baking potatoes
2   tablespoons hot water
1   tablespoon instant tea
½   cup sour cream
¼   cup finely chopped onion
1   tablespoon chives
1   teaspoon salt
       Pinch black pepper
⅔   cup cubed Velveeta cheese

THIS RECIPE

is LOW in HEME iron and contains the following substances that inhibit absorption of nonheme iron:

✓ calcium

✓ dairy phosphate

eggs

✓ phytate phosphorus

POLYPHENOLS

✓ tannic acid

✓ chlorogenic acid

phenolic acid

✓ oxalates

PER SERVING

IRON	heme iron	nonheme iron
	0.0 mg	1.1 mg

Wash the potatoes and bake at 350° for 1 hour.

Remove, cool, and cut off the top, creating a shoe. Scoop out the potato meat and place in a bowl.

In a separate bowl mix the water and tea, and stir in the sour cream. Blend well. Add the sour cream mixture, onion, chives, salt, pepper, and Velveeta to the potato meat. Combine well and spoon back into the shells. Cover loosely and rebake uncovered at 300° for about 30 to 40 minutes.

Let stand 10 to 15 minutes before serving.

Serves 4

Carol's Sweet Onion Casserole

6 cups coarsely chopped sweet onion (Vidalia)

4 cups shredded Swiss cheese

2 cups Hellman's brand mayonnaise

¼ cup Parmesan cheese

This Recipe

is LOW in HEME iron and contains the following substances that inhibit absorption of nonheme iron:

✓ calcium

dairy phosphate

eggs

phytate phosphorus

POLYPHENOLS

tannic acid

chlorogenic acid

phenolic acid

oxalates

Per Serving

IRON	heme iron	nonheme iron
	0.0 mg	0.2 mg

Preheat oven to 350 degrees.

Remove onion skins; cut into chunks and chop in a food processor. Dump chopped onions into a large mixing bowl. Add Swiss cheese and mayonnaise. Blend together until well mixed. Pour mixture into a 13x9 ungreased baking dish. Sprinkle Parmesan cheese on top. Bake covered at 350 degrees for 1 hour then, uncovered for 15 to 20 minutes or until top is browned and bubbly. Let stand 15 minutes before serving.

This rich but delicious dish, submitted by Carol Bates of Atlanta, Georgia, is a family favorite we all look forward to each Fourth of July when Vidalia onions are plentiful. For fat-restricted diets, Hellman's lowfat mayonnaise may be substituted.

Sauces

Sauces provide body and taste to recipes. When made in the traditional way with butter and cream, sauces undoubtedly add calories and animal fat to a recipe. Eliminating sauces from one's diet is not necessary. For persons who are in good health, exercise regularly, and incorporate variety into their diet, traditional butter and cream sauces can be enjoyed from time to time. For those who must reduce the amount of animal fat in their diet or reduce both fat and calories, reducing the consumption of rich sauces is one way to achieve this diet goal.

Most sauces are made with a combination of fat and flour, called a roux, to which broth is added. The roux mixture thickens the sauce, although some cooks use cornstarch as a thickening agent, especially for oriental recipes or fruit desserts. In the *Hemochromatosis Cookbook* a roux using olive oil as the fat in combination with oat blend, whole-wheat, rice bran, barley, soy, or buckwheat flour provides a healthy basis for sauces and gravies. Olive oil is rich in monounsaturated fat, the type that contributes to good health. Whole-grain flours are an excellent source of phytate, which impairs iron absorption.

Some sauces can be made with low-fat mayonnaise and sour cream substitutes. reduced-fat mayonnaise and reduced-fat sour cream are available commercially. Hellman's makes an excellent reduced-fat mayonnaise. Breakstone makes an excellent reduced-fat sour cream. Since tastes vary within families, sometimes it is more economical to make your own blends; below are some easy reduced-fat recipes:

Reduced-fat sour cream: Mix plain yogurt with regular sour cream 2:1. This reduces the amount of fat while maintaining the flavor and texture of sour cream.

Reduced-fat mayonnaise #1: In a blender mix 1 cup Hellman's brand mayonnaise and ¼ cup brewed tea. Tea will discolor mayo but not change the taste significantly. Refrigerate to thicken.

Reduced-fat mayo spread #2: In a blender combine ½ cup Hellman's brand mayonnaise, ¼ cup spicy mustard, ⅓ cup liquid lecithin, 1¼ teaspoons balsamic vinegar, 1 teaspoon of instant tea, ¼ to ½ teaspoon of salt, and ⅓ cup of olive oil. Combine all ingredients in a blender. Refrigerate to thicken. *Note: Lecithin when taken daily can help reduce LDL cholesterol. Lecithin has a strong taste and will cause the spread to have a yellow color. Herbs such as basil, oregano, marjoram, chives, chervil, etc., can be added to this spread to give it extra zest.*

Barbecue Sauce

4 tablespoons olive oil
1½ cups finely chopped onion
4 tablespoons minced garlic
1 6-ounce can tomato paste
3 cans hot strong black coffee
1 cup Heinz ketchup
½ cup apple cider vinegar
1½ cups firmly packed brown sugar
4 tablespoons spicy mustard
½ teaspoon red pepper

In a stockpot heat the oil and sauté the onion and garlic until tender and golden, about 20 minutes.

Add the remaining ingredients and simmer for 1 hour.

Refrigerate and use as needed.

Makes 4½ to 5 cups
Serving size: 2 tablespoons

THIS RECIPE

is LOW in HEME iron and contains the following substances that inhibit absorption of nonheme iron:

calcium

dairy phosphate

eggs

phytate phosphorus

POLYPHENOLS

✓ tannic acid

✓ chlorogenic acid

phenolic acid

oxalates

PER SERVING

IRON	heme iron	nonheme iron
	0.0 mg	0.3 mg

Brown Sauce

½   cup olive oil
2   cups finely chopped onions
S   Salt and pepper to taste
½   cup flour
4   cups stock
1   cup brewed strong black coffee
1   stalk celery, chopped
1   parsnip, chopped
¼   cup tomato sauce
2   tablespoons chopped fresh parsley
1   tablespoon minced garlic
¼   teaspoon thyme
1   bay leaf

In a skillet heat the oil and sauté the onion until tender and beginning to brown, about 20 minutes.

Season the onion with salt and pepper. Whisk the flour into the onion. Gently pour in the stock. Add the coffee, celery, parsnip, and tomato sauce. Add the parsley, garlic, thyme, and bay leaf. Simmer until reduced to a thick sauce.

Remove the bay leaf before serving.

Makes 6 cups; serving size: ½ cup

THIS RECIPE

is LOW in HEME iron and contains the following substances that inhibit absorption of nonheme iron:

calcium	
✓ dairy phosphate	
eggs	
✓ phytate phosphorus	
POLYPHENOLS	
✓ tannic acid	
✓ chlorogenic acid	
phenolic acid	
oxalates	

PER SERVING

IRON	heme iron	nonheme iron
	trace	0.2 mg

Cheese Sauce

2 tablespoons olive oil (or butter)
4 tablespoons flour
1 teaspoon salt
¼ teaspoon white pepper
1¼ cups lowfat milk

FOR BASIC AMERICAN MACARONI AND CHEESE SAUCE:
½ cup cubed Velveeta cheese
½ cup shredded sharp Cheddar cheese

FOR MORNAY:
1 cup shredded Swiss cheese

FOR ALFREDO:
Substitute cream for milk
1 cup grated Parmesan or Romano cheese

In a skillet heat the oil. Whisk in the flour, salt, and pepper, and continue whisking until a paste forms. Very slowly add the milk, stirring until smooth. Season with salt and pepper. Blend in the cheeses as desired.

Other cheese choices include: mozzarella, havarti, fontina, Neufchâtel, Monterey Jack, etc.

Note: Some cheeses melt better than others; combinations of cheeses can provide a better textured sauce.

Serving size: ¼ cup

THIS RECIPE

is LOW in HEME iron and contains the following substances that inhibit absorption of nonheme iron:

✓ calcium
✓ dairy phosphate
eggs
phytate phosphorus
POLYPHENOLS
tannic acid
chlorogenic acid
phenolic acid
oxalates

PER SERVING

IRON	heme iron	nonheme iron
	trace	0.2 mg

Cream Sauce with Roasted Peppers

1   medium red bell pepper
1   cup milk
2   tablespoons olive oil
4   tablespoons flour
1   teaspoon salt
¼   teaspoon white pepper
½   cup heavy cream

THIS RECIPE

*is LOW in HEME iron and contains
the following substances that
inhibit absorption of nonheme iron:*

✓ calcium

✓ dairy phosphate

eggs

✓ phytate phosphorus

polyphenols

tannic acid

chlorogenic acid

phenolic acid

oxalates

PER SERVING

IRON	heme iron	nonheme iron
	0.0 mg	0.2 mg

Wash the pepper, remove the seeds and stem. Brush the pepper with olive oil and cut into slivers. Roast under the broiler for about 5 to 7 minutes.

Pour the milk into a food processor. Add the roasted peppers and blend. Prepare the roux: In a saucepan heat the olive oil. Blend in the flour until smooth. Slowly pour in the milk, blending until smooth. Season with salt and pepper. Add the heavy cream and reheat the sauce. It is delicious served over fish or vegetables.

Makes 1½ cups
Serving size: ¼ cup

Chicken Velouté

2 tablespoons olive oil
¼ cup flour
1 teaspoon salt
¼ teaspoon white pepper
½ cup brewed coffee
1½ cups chicken broth
¼ cup finely diced chicken (white meat)

In a skillet or saucepan heat the olive oil. Whisk in the flour, blending until smooth. Add salt and pepper, and stir until light brown. Slowly add the coffee and chicken broth. Add the chicken.

Makes 2¼ cups or 6 servings

THIS RECIPE

is LOW in HEME iron and contains the following substances that inhibit absorption of nonheme iron:

	calcium
	✓ dairy phosphate
	eggs
	✓ phytate phosphorus
	POLYPHENOLS
THIS RECIPE	✓ tannic acid
	✓ chlorogenic acid
	phenolic acid
	oxalates

PER SERVING

IRON	heme iron	nonheme iron
	0.03 mg	0.4 mg

Gravy

2 tablespoons olive oil
¼ cup flour
1 teaspoon salt
¼ teaspoon black pepper
1½ cups chicken or turkey broth
½ cup coffee
1 teaspoon instant coffee

In a skillet or saucepan heat the oil. Whisk in the flour, blending until smooth. Add the salt and pepper. Slowly add the broth and coffee, blending well.

For white gravy omit the instant coffee and add ¼ cup of milk.

Makes 2¼ cups or 6 to 8 servings

THIS RECIPE

is LOW in HEME iron and contains the following substances that inhibit absorption of nonheme iron:

✓ calcium

✓ dairy phosphate

eggs

✓ phytate phosphorus

POLYPHENOLS

✓ tannic acid

THIS RECIPE

✓ chlorogenic acid

phenolic acid

oxalates

PER SERVING

IRON	heme iron	nonheme iron
	0.26 mg	0.5 mg

Gumbo

¼ cup olive oil
2 cups chopped onion
1 cup diced celery, stems included
4 cups diced tomatoes
8 cups turkey or chicken broth
½ cup chopped fresh parsley
1 tablespoon instant coffee
2 bay leaves
1 tablespoon basil
1 tablespoon thyme
2 tablespoons minced garlic
1 tablespoon salt
   Red pepper to taste
¼ cup olive oil
½ cup flour

In a skillet heat ¼ cup of olive oil and sauté the onion for about 20 minutes.

Add the celery and cook until tender. Add the tomatoes and cook an additional 20 minutes. Add the broth, parsley, instant coffee, bay leaves, basil, thyme, garlic, salt, and red pepper.

Prepare a roux: In a saucepan heat ¼ cup of olive oil. Add ½ cup of flour slowly, whisking into a paste. Continue cooking until the paste turns brown, but take care not to burn the roux. The next step is a bit tricky, so wear oven mitts to protect arms from splatter. Dip a cupful of liquid from the soup and add cautiously to the paste. Whisk constantly; continue to add cupfuls of soup to the paste until it is a gravy-like consistency. Whisk the gravy back into the soup. The soup will take on a cloudy appearance and will thicken slightly. Remove the bay leaves before serving.

Gumbo can be served over beans and rice and topped with chopped green onion.

Serves 6

THIS RECIPE

is LOW in HEME iron and contains the following substances that inhibit absorption of nonheme iron:

calcium
✓ dairy phosphate
eggs
✓ phytate phosphorus
POLYPHENOLS
✓ tannic acid
✓ chlorogenic acid
phenolic acid
oxalates

PER SERVING

IRON	heme iron	nonheme iron
	trace	0.56 mg

Marinara Sauce

¼ cup olive oil
4 cups finely chopped onion
¼ cup minced garlic
1 14.5-ounce can diced tomatoes or 1 cup fresh
1 28-ounce can crushed tomatoes with purée
1 6-ounce can tomato paste
2 6-ounce cans hot coffee
1 cup chopped fresh parsley
1 teaspoon salt
Red pepper to taste

In a saucepan heat the olive oil and sauté the onion and garlic for 20 minutes.

Add the diced tomatoes and simmer until the tomatoes are tender.

Add the tomato purée, tomato paste, and hot coffee. Add the parsley, and season with salt and pepper. Cover and simmer for 1 hour.

Uncover and simmer for 30 minutes.

Makes 8 cups
Serving size: 1 cup

THIS RECIPE

is LOW in HEME iron and contains the following substances that inhibit absorption of nonheme iron:

calcium
✓ dairy phosphate
eggs
✓ phytate phosphorus
POLYPHENOLS
✓ tannic acid
✓ chlorogenic acid
phenolic acid
oxalates

PER SERVING

IRON	heme iron	nonheme iron
	0.0 mg	0.58 mg

Mushroom Velouté

2 tablespoons olive oil
¼ cup diced mushrooms
¼ cup oat flour
1 teaspoon salt
¼ teaspoon white pepper
1½ cups vegetable broth
½ cup brewed tea

In skillet or saucepan heat the olive oil and sauté the mushrooms until tender. Whisk in the flour, salt, and pepper. As the mixture turns brown, slowly add the broth and tea. Continue whisking until the mixture thickens.

Makes 4 cups
Serving size: ¼ cup

THIS RECIPE

is LOW in HEME iron and contains the following substances that inhibit absorption of nonheme iron:

calcium

dairy phosphate

eggs

✓ phytate phosphorus

POLYPHENOLS

✓ tannic acid

chlorogenic acid

phenolic acid

oxalates

PER SERVING

IRON	heme iron	nonheme iron
	trace	0.28 mg

The Hemochromatosis Cookbook

Rosemary Sour Cream Sauce

2 tablespoons butter
2 tablespoons olive oil
2 tablespoons fresh or dried rosemary
2 tablespoons chives
1 cup sour cream

In a saucepan melt the butter. Add the oil, herbs, and sour cream. Whisk together and heat through but do not boil.

Best served with potatoes, vegetables, or fish.

Serves 4

THIS RECIPE

is LOW in HEME iron and contains the following substances that inhibit absorption of nonheme iron:

✓ calcium

✓ dairy phosphate

eggs

phytate phosphorus

POLYPHENOLS

tannic acid

chlorogenic acid

phenolic acid

✓ oxalates

PER SERVING

IRON	heme iron	nonheme iron
	trace	trace

Roux

2 tablespoons olive oil
4 tablespoons flour
1 teaspoon salt
⅛ teaspoon white pepper

PER SERVING

IRON	heme iron	nonheme iron
	trace	0.7 mg

In a glass skillet heat the oil. Whisk in the flour and continue whisking until a paste forms and begins to darken. Season with salt and pepper.

From this roux the following recipes can be made: white sauce, cream sauce, gravy, cheese sauces, veloutés, and cream-based soups.

Serves 4

Sweet-and-Sour Sauce

1 tablespoon olive oil
1 cup green bell pepper cut into julienne strips
½ cup soy sauce
½ cup brown sugar
½ cup pineapple juice
½ teaspoon ground ginger root
1 tablespoon instant coffee
¼ cup water
2 teaspoons cornstarch

In a saucepan heat the oil and sauté the peppers until tender. Remove from the skillet and set aside.

In the same skillet combine the soy sauce, brown sugar, pineapple juice, ginger root, and coffee, and bring to a boil.

In a shaker container mix the water and cornstarch; shake vigorously. Using a whisk, stir the sauce briskly and add the cornstarch-water mixture to the boiling sauce whisking constantly. The sauce should thicken slightly.

Makes about 2 cups
Serving size: ¼ cup

THIS RECIPE

is LOW in HEME iron and contains the following substances that inhibit absorption of nonheme iron:

calcium
✓ dairy phosphate
eggs
✓ phytate phosphorus
POLYPHENOLS
✓ tannic acid
✓ chlorogenic acid
phenolic acid
oxalates

PER SERVING

IRON	heme iron	nonheme iron
	trace	1.0 mg

Vegetable Velouté

2   tablespoons olive oil
1/4   cup finely diced vegetable of choice: celery, onion or leeks, parsnips, spinach, kale, carrot, red, green, or yellow peppers
1/4   cup flour
1   teaspoon salt
1/4   teaspoon white pepper
1 1/2   cups vegetable broth
1/2   cup brewed tea
1/2   cup heavy cream

In skillet or saucepan heat the olive oil. Add the desired vegetable and sauté until tender. Whisk in the flour. Season with salt and pepper. Stir until light brown. Slowly add the broth, tea, and cream and blend until smooth.

Makes 2 1/4 cups or 6 servings

THIS RECIPE

is LOW in HEME iron and contains the following substances that inhibit absorption of nonheme iron:

calcium
✓ dairy phosphate
eggs

THIS RECIPE

✓ phytate phosphorus

POLYPHENOLS
✓ tannic acid
chlorogenic acid
phenolic acid
✓ oxalates

PER SERVING

IRON	heme iron	nonheme iron
	0.0 mg	0.4 mg

White Sauce

2   tablespoons olive oil
4   tablespoons flour
1   teaspoon salt
¼   teaspoon white pepper
1¼ cups lowfat milk

In a saucepan heat the olive oil and blend in the flour. Season with salt and pepper. Very slowly add the milk, blending well.

Makes 1½ cups
Serving size: ¼ cup

THIS RECIPE

is LOW in HEME iron and contains the following substances that inhibit absorption of nonheme iron:

✓ calcium
✓ dairy phosphate
eggs
✓ phytate phosphorus
POLYPHENOLS
tannic acid
chlorogenic acid
phenolic acid
oxalates

PER SERVING

IRON	heme iron	nonheme iron
	0.0 mg	0.12 mg

Apple Oatmeal Cookies

1	cup chopped seeded apples
2	tablespoons apple juice
1/2	cup butter
2/3	cup light brown sugar
2	eggs
1	cup oat blend flour
1	teaspoon baking powder
1	teaspoon cinnamon
1/2	teaspoon nutmeg
1/2	teaspoon salt
1	cup oats
1	cup English walnuts

In a food processor place the apples and apple juice, and pulse until the apples are coarse chunks.

In a separate bowl cream the butter and sugar. Add the eggs and blend well. Sift the flour, baking powder, cinnamon, nutmeg, and salt into the mixture. Stir in the oats and apples, and mix well. Fold in the nuts. Spoon onto a greased baking sheet. Bake at 350° for 10 to 15 minutes.

Makes 2 dozen

This Recipe

is LOW in HEME iron and contains the following substances that inhibit absorption of nonheme iron:

calcium

✓ dairy phosphate

✓ eggs

✓ phytate phosphorus

POLYPHENOLS

✓ tannic acid

✓ chlorogenic acid

✓ phenolic acid

oxalates

Per Serving

IRON	heme iron	nonheme iron
	0.0 mg	0.2 mg

Baked Dutch Apple Pie

8   peeled, seeded, and sliced cooking apples
1½   tablespoons apple juice
⅔   cup light brown sugar, firmly packed
¼   teaspoon salt
¼   cup oat blend flour
1   teaspoon ground cinnamon
1   tablespoon instant tea
½   teaspoon ground nutmeg
1   9-inch pie crust

TOPPING:
1   cup flour
⅔   cup firmly packed light brown sugar
½   cup butter, melted

Preheat the oven to 350°.

In a large bowl combine the apples, apple juice, ⅔ cup of brown sugar, salt, ¼ cup of flour, cinnamon, instant tea, and nutmeg. Mix the ingredients well, then spoon into the crust.

Prepare the topping: In a separate bowl combine with a fork 1 cup of flour, ⅔ cup of brown sugar, and ½ cup of butter. Sprinkle the topping mixture evenly over the apples. Place the pie on a baking sheet and bake for about 55 to 60 minutes until the topping is golden and the filling bubbles.

Serves 8

THIS RECIPE

is LOW in HEME iron and contains the following substances that inhibit absorption of nonheme iron:

✓ calcium
✓ dairy phosphate
✓ eggs
✓ phytate phosphorus
POLYPHENOLS
✓ tannic acid
✓ chlorogenic acid
✓ phenolic acid
oxalates

PER SERVING

IRON	heme iron	nonheme iron
	0.0 mg	1.1 mg

The Hemochromatosis Cookbook

Banana Pudding

1   12-ounce box vanilla wafers
4   large bananas
2½   cups cold milk
½   cup chilled tea
1   4-ounce package Jello-O brand
       instant vanilla pudding mix
       Whipped topping of your choice

In a large bowl alternate layers of vanilla wafers and sliced bananas.

In a separate bowl mix the milk, tea, and pudding with a wire whisk. Work quickly so the mixture does not thicken before pouring over the bananas. Top with whipped cream or nondairy topping.

Serves 8

THIS RECIPE

is LOW in HEME iron and contains the following substances that inhibit absorption of nonheme iron:

✓ calcium

✓ dairy phosphate

eggs

✓ phytate phosphorus

POLYPHENOLS

✓ tannic acid

THIS RECIPE   ✓ chlorogenic acid

phenolic acid

oxalates

PER SERVING

IRON	heme iron	nonheme iron
	0.0 mg	0.5 mg

Buttermilk Sheet Cake

3/4   cup butter
2   cups light brown sugar
2   eggs
1   teaspoon vanilla extract
1   teaspoon baking soda
1¼   cups buttermilk
2¾   cups flour
1   teaspoon baking powder
¼   teaspoon salt
1   heaping teaspoon cinnamon

TOPPING:
2   egg whites
1   cup light brown sugar
½   cup walnuts

In a large bowl cream the butter and 2 cups of brown sugar together. Add the 2 eggs and beat well. Add the vanilla.

Sprinkle the baking soda into the buttermilk and set aside.

In a separate bowl mix the flour, baking powder, salt, and cinnamon. Alternate adding the dry ingredients and buttermilk to the creamed mixture. stirring with a wooden spoon.

Oil and flour a 9 x 13-inch baking dish. Pour the cake batter into the dish.

Prepare the topping: In the bowl of an electric mixer beat 2 egg whites until soft peaks form. Slowly fold the whites into 1 cup of light brown sugar. Add the English walnuts. Spoon evenly over the cake batter. Bake at 325° for 40 minutes.

Serves 12

THIS RECIPE

is LOW in HEME iron and contains the following substances that inhibit absorption of nonheme iron:

calcium
✓ dairy phosphate
✓ eggs
✓ phytate phosphorus
POLYPHENOLS
✓ tannic acid
✓ chlorogenic acid
phenolic acid
oxalates

PER SERVING

IRON	heme iron	nonheme iron
	0.0 mg	1.3 mg

Chess Pie

2 cups firmly packed light brown sugar
1 tablespoon oat blend flour
1 tablespoon Yelton's brand cornmeal
1 teaspoon cinnamon
¼ teaspoon salt
¼ cup olive oil
½ cup apple juice
½ cup light cream
1 teaspoon instant tea
4 eggs, lightly beaten
1 9-inch unbaked pie shell

In a large bowl mix the sugar, flour, cornmeal, cinnamon, and salt. Add the oil, juice, cream, and tea, and blend well. Add the eggs and blend well. Pour the mixture into the unbaked pie shell. Bake at 350° for 40 minutes.

Serves 8

THIS RECIPE

is LOW in HEME iron and contains the following substances that inhibit absorption of nonheme iron:

✓ calcium
✓ dairy phosphate
✓ eggs
✓ phytate phosphorus

POLYPHENOLS

✓ tannic acid
✓ chlorogenic acid
phenolic acid
oxalates

PER SERVING

IRON	heme iron	nonheme iron
	0.0 mg	1.36 mg

Coffee Liqueur Chocolate Cake

1   18¼-ounce box Duncan Hines devil's food cake mix

1   4-ounce package Jell-O brand instant chocolate pudding

½   cup strong coffee

½   cup Faux Molasses (see page 258)

1   cup buttermilk

¼   teaspoon baking soda

½   cup olive oil

4   eggs

1   6-ounce bag semisweet chocolate bits

Spray the inside of a bundt cake pan generously with vegetable spray.

In a large bowl blend all of the ingredients, folding in the chocolate chips last. Pour the batter evenly into the prepared bundt pan. Bake at 350° for 40 minutes.

Serves 8

THIS RECIPE

is LOW in HEME iron and contains the following substances that inhibit absorption of nonheme iron:

✓ calcium

✓ dairy phosphate

✓ eggs

✓ phytate phosphorus

POLYPHENOLS

✓ tannic acid

✓ chlorogenic acid

phenolic acid

oxalates

PER SERVING

IRON	heme iron	nonheme iron
	0.0 mg	0.47 mg

Custard Apple Pie

1   9-inch pie crust
3   cups peeled, seeded, and diced Granny Smith apples
2   tablespoons apple juice (to retard discoloration)
2   tablespoons olive oil
1   teaspoon cinnamon
1   egg
1   14-ounce can sweetened condensed milk

Preheat the oven to 375°. Bake the pie crust for 5 to 7 minutes until light brown.

In a saucepan simmer the apples, apple juice, oil, and cinnamon on low heat until the apples are tender and the liquid evaporates. Mash the cooked apples into coarse applesauce and pour into the baked pie crust. In a medium bowl beat the egg into the condensed milk. Pour over the apples. Bake at 350° for 40 minutes.

Serves 8

THIS RECIPE

is LOW in HEME iron and contains the following substances that inhibit absorption of nonheme iron:

✓ calcium

✓ dairy phosphate

✓ eggs

✓ phytate phosphorus

POLYPHENOLS

✓ tannic acid

✓ chlorogenic acid

✓ phenolic acid

oxalates

PER SERVING

IRON	heme iron	nonheme iron
	0.0 mg	0.25 mg

Faux Molasses

2 cups firmly packed brown sugar
1 cup water
2 tablespoons instant decaffeinated coffee

In a saucepan combine all of the ingredients. Bring to a boil. Allow to boil for 5 minutes.

Remove the pan from the heat and let stand until thickened.

Makes 1½ cups

THIS RECIPE

is LOW in HEME iron and contains the following substances that inhibit absorption of nonheme iron:

✓ calcium

dairy phosphate

eggs

phytate phosphorus

POLYPHENOLS

✓ tannic acid

✓ chlorogenic acid

phenolic acid

oxalates

THIS RECIPE
PER SERVING

IRON	heme iron	nonheme iron
	0.0 mg	1.4 mg

Ice Cream Cake

THIS RECIPE

*is LOW in HEME iron and contains
the following substances that
inhibit absorption of nonheme iron:*

✓ calcium

✓ dairy phosphate

✓ eggs

✓ phytate phosphorus

POLYPHENOLS

✓ tannic acid

✓ chlorogenic acid

phenolic acid

oxalates

PER SERVING

IRON	heme iron	nonheme iron
	0.0 mg	0.7 mg

Prepare 1 store-bought chocolate brownie recipe in one 9-inch round cake pan.

Let ½ gallon Breyer's brand coffee ice cream soften for 30 minutes or longer to thaw slightly.

Empty the ice cream into a 9-inch cake pan and press firmly, distributing the ice cream evenly. Refreeze overnight.

Thaw 1 tub of whipped topping overnight.

To assemble: Place the baked and cooled brownie on a flat dinner plate. Fill the kitchen sink with 4 to 6 inches of warm water. Holding the cake pan with frozen ice cream, carefully submerge the pan up to the rim in the warm water. Take care not to allow the water to splash onto the ice cream. Gently move the pan back and forth until the frozen contents loosen. Place the cake layer on top of the frozen ice cream. Secure the cake with one hand and the ice cream pan with the other hand. Flip both the cake and pan over so the cake is on the bottom and the pan can be removed from the ice cream layer now on top. Slide the cake onto a flat dish. Place the cake in the freezer for 1 hour.

Frost the cake with whipped topping.

Tip: Frozen yogurt or ice milk can be substituted.

Serves 8 to 10

Lime Jell-O Salad

1   cup hot tea
1   6-ounce box lime Jell-O
1   8-ounce package Neufchâtel
     cream cheese
1   cup cold apple juice
½   cup chopped apples
¼   cup chopped celery
½   cup chopped English walnuts
     Sour cream for topping

In a large bowl pour the hot tea over the gelatin and stir until completely dissolved. Add the Neufchâtel and mix until the cheese is blended. Add the cold apple juice, apples, celery, and nuts. Stir and pour into a sprayed mold or glass dish. Refrigerate until set.

Serve with a dollop of sour cream.

Serves 8

THIS RECIPE

*is LOW in HEME iron and contains
the following substances that
inhibit absorption of nonheme iron:*

✓ calcium

✓ dairy phosphate

eggs

✓ phytate phosphorus

POLYPHENOLS

✓ tannic acid

✓ chlorogenic acid

phenolic acid

oxalates

PER SERVING

IRON	heme iron	nonheme iron
	0.0 mg	0.3 mg

Mocha Almond Biscotti

2½ cups raw almonds
3 cups oat blend flour
¼ cup cocoa
1 tablespoon instant coffee
2½ teaspoons baking powder
¼ teaspoon salt
½ cup butter
1 cup sugar
3 eggs
1 teaspoon vanilla extract
1 teaspoon almond extract

THIS RECIPE

is LOW in HEME iron and contains the following substances that inhibit absorption of nonheme iron:

✓ calcium
✓ dairy phosphate
✓ eggs
✓ phytate phosphorus
POLYPHENOLS
✓ tannic acid
✓ chlorogenic acid
phenolic acid
oxalates

PER SERVING

IRON	heme iron	nonheme iron
	trace	0.95 mg

Place the raw almonds on a cookie sheet and roast at 425° for 15 minutes. Remove from the oven and let stand 20 minutes or until crunchy. Chop in a food processor.

In a medium bowl combine the flour, cocoa, instant coffee, baking powder, and salt.

In the bowl of an electric mixer cream the butter and sugar together. Add the eggs and continue to beat at medium speed. Add the dry ingredients. Blend in the vanilla and almond extracts and the nuts. Blend well, the dough will be stiff. Turn dough out onto a floured pastry cloth. Form into 2 long oval-shaped flattened logs. Place on a cookie sheet. Bake at 350° for about 20 minutes.

Transfer to a cool surface and cut the logs widthwise into 1½-inch-wide pieces. Place the pieces on their sides on the cookie sheet and bake at 400° for 10 minutes.

Makes 18

Mocha Angel Food

1¼ cups sifted cake flour
2   tablespoons instant coffee
3   tablespoons cocoa
12 large egg whites (let stand to reach room temperature)
1½ teaspoons cream of tartar
¼   teaspoon salt
1   cup sugar
1   teaspoon vanilla extract

CHOCOLATE-COFFEE SAUCE:
(*Optional—not recommended for diabetics*)
¾   cup sweetened condensed milk
½   cup semisweet chocolate bits
2   tablespoons instant coffee

THIS RECIPE

*is LOW in HEME iron and contains
the following substances that
inhibit absorption of nonheme iron:*

✓ calcium
✓ dairy phosphate
✓ eggs
✓ phytate phosphorus
POLYPHENOLS
✓ tannic acid
✓ chlorogenic acid
phenolic acid
oxalates

PER SERVING

IRON	heme iron	nonheme iron
	0.0 mg	0.7 mg

Place the oven rack on the lowest level and preheat the oven to 350°.

In a medium bowl sift the flour, coffee, and cocoa powder together 4 times and set aside.

In the bowl of an electric mixer beat the egg whites until foamy. Add the cream of tartar and salt. Turn the mixer to low speed and alternately add the sugar and flour mixture in small amounts to the whipped egg white mixture. Drizzle in the vanilla. Pour into a nonstick angel food cake pan. Bake at 350° for 40 to 45 minutes or until the cake springs back upon touch.

Invert the pan onto a cooling rack and let stand to cool.

To make the sauce, in a medium saucepan heat the condensed milk. Add the chocolate bits and coffee, and whip with a whisk until smooth and creamy. While warm, drizzle over the top of the cake.

Serves 8

Mocha Cheesecake

CRUST:

1½ cups graham cracker crumbs

⅓ cup brown sugar

⅓ cup olive oil

FILLING:

4 8-ounce packages cream cheese

1 cup sugar

3 tablespoons flour

½ cup Hershey's brand cocoa

1 tablespoon instant coffee

1¼ cups sour cream

2 teaspoons vanilla extract

4 eggs

TOPPING:

½ cup sour cream

1 tablespoon milk

Cocoa powder for garnish

In a medium bowl blend together the graham cracker crumbs, brown sugar, and olive oil. Press into the bottom of a 10-inch springform pan.

In the bowl of an electric mixer combine the cream cheese, sugar, flour, cocoa, and coffee. Beat until fluffy. Add the sour cream and vanilla, then eggs one at a time. Blend well on low speed. Pour into the graham cracker crust. Bake at 300° for 1 hour. Cool.

In a small bowl combine the sour cream and milk. Pour over the top of the cheesecake. Cool the cheesecake in the refrigerator overnight, or at least 6 hours before removing the outside ring.

Slide a thin-blade knife between the cheesecake and the bottom of the pan. Slip the cheesecake onto a glass plate. Garnish with sprinkle of cocoa powder.

Serves 12

THIS RECIPE

*is LOW in HEME iron and contains
the following substances that
inhibit absorption of nonheme iron:*

✓ calcium

✓ dairy phosphate

✓ eggs

✓ phytate phosphorus

POLYPHENOLS

✓ tannic acid

✓ chlorogenic acid

phenolic acid

oxalates

PER SERVING

IRON	heme iron	nonheme iron
	0.0 mg	0.9 mg

Mocha Cream Pie

½ cup sugar
5 egg yolks
1 cup milk
3 ounces semisweet chocolate
1 ounce unsweetened chocolate
1 tablespoon instant coffee
1½ packets unflavored gelatin
1 tablespoon cold coffee
1 cup heavy cream
1 9-inch pie shell, baked

THIS RECIPE

*is LOW in HEME iron and contains
the following substances that
inhibit absorption of nonheme iron:*

✓ calcium
✓ dairy phosphate
✓ eggs
✓ phytate phosphorus
POLYPHENOLS
✓ tannic acid
✓ chlorogenic acid
phenolic acid
oxalates

PER SERVING

IRON	heme iron	nonheme iron
	0.0 mg	1.0 mg

In the bowl of an electric mixer combine the sugar and egg yolks. Beat on high until the mixture is pale lemon-colored.

In a saucepan heat the milk on medium low. Add the chocolate squares and instant coffee and stir until melted and smooth.

In a separate bowl dissolve the gelatin with cold coffee. Blend the gelatin into the warm milk-chocolate mixture and stir with a wooden spoon for about 5 to 7 minutes. Begin adding the egg-sugar mixture to the chocolate mixture. Stir quickly so the egg does not cook. Once blended, pour the mixture into a large bowl and set the bottom of the bowl into an ice water bath. Stir until the mixture thickens. Whip the cream until soft peaks form. Fold into the chocolate pudding. Blend thoroughly. Pour into the baked pie crust. Refrigerate.

Serves 6

Mocha Nut Triangles

2¼ cups ground English walnuts
2   cups confectioners' sugar
2   tablespoons Folger's brand instant decaf coffee
2   tablespoons brewed hot decaf coffee
½   cup semisweet chocolate bits

THIS RECIPE

is LOW in HEME iron and contains the following substances that inhibit absorption of nonheme iron:

	calcium
✓	dairy phosphate
	eggs
✓	phytate phosphorus
	POLYPHENOLS
✓	tannic acid
✓	chlorogenic acid
	phenolic acid
	oxalates

PER SERVING

IRON	heme iron	nonheme iron
	0.0 mg	0.8 mg

In a medium bowl combine 2 cups of nuts and 1¾ cups of the confectioners' sugar. Stir in 1 tablespoon of instant coffee and add 1 tablespoon of the hot brewed coffee. Work the mixture into a ball and refrigerate overnight.

Sift confectioners' sugar onto the surface of the ball and roll out on a clean flat surface. Cut into wide strips, and score each strip to create rectangles. Cut each rectangle on the diagonal to create triangles.

In the top of a double boiler over simmering water melt the chocolate bits. Add ¼ cup of confectioners' sugar. Add the remaining 1 tablespoon of instant coffee and 1 tablespoon of brewed coffee, and stir until the chocolate is silky. Spoon the chocolate over the triangles. Decorate with a pinch of ground nuts.

Makes 1 pound

Mocha Tiramisu

12 ladyfingers
3   cups milk
⅔   cup sugar
¼   teaspoon salt
2   tablespoons instant coffee granules
2   packets unflavored gelatin
¼   cup brewed cold coffee
¼   cup Faux Molasses (see recipe on page 258)
2   cups heavy cream

THIS RECIPE

is LOW in HEME iron and contains the following substances that inhibit absorption of nonheme iron:

✓ calcium
✓ dairy phosphate
eggs
✓ phytate phosphorus
POLYPHENOLS
✓ tannic acid
✓ chlorogenic acid
phenolic acid
oxalates

PER SERVING

IRON	heme iron	nonheme iron
	0.0 mg	trace

Line the sides of a large straight glass bowl with ladyfingers.

In a glass saucepan heat the milk over medium-low heat. Add the sugar, salt, and instant coffee granules to the warm milk. In a separate bowl dissolve the gelatin in cold coffee. When dissolved, add the gelatin mixture to the warm milk mixture and stir with a wooden spoon for about 5 to 7 minutes until the pudding thickens. Add the Faux Molasses to the pudding and chill slightly.

In the bowl of an electric mixer whip the cream until soft peaks form. Fold into the pudding. Pour the mixture into the center of the ladyfinger-lined bowl. Refrigerate.

Serves 12

Peanut Butter Cookies

1 cup sugar

1 cup firmly packed light brown sugar

½ cup olive oil

1 cup Jif brand chunky peanut butter

2 eggs

1 teaspoon vanilla extract

2½ to 3 cups flour

1 teaspoon baking soda

1 teaspoon salt

In a large bowl cream together the sugars, oil, and peanut butter. Add the eggs and vanilla.

In a separate bowl sift together the flour, baking soda, and salt. Add slowly to the sugar mixture. The dough will be stiff as the flour is worked into it. When all sides of the bowl are clean, using an ice cream scoop with a release handle, scoop the dough onto a lightly oiled cookie sheet. Mash each cookie and make a criss-cross design on top using the tines of a dinner fork. Bake at 350° for 6 to 8 minutes or until brown around the edges.

Makes 24 cookies

THIS RECIPE

is LOW in HEME iron and contains the following substances that inhibit absorption of nonheme iron:

✓ calcium

✓ dairy phosphate

✓ eggs

✓ phytate phosphorus

POLYPHENOLS

✓ tannic acid

chlorogenic acid

phenolic acid

oxalates

PER SERVING

IRON	heme iron	nonheme iron
	0.0 mg	0.5 mg

Peanut Butter Chocolate Ice Cream Pie

1 8-ounce package Neufchâtel cheese
1¼ cups confectioners' sugar
1 cup crunchy Jif brand peanut butter
2 cups light cream
2 tablespoons Hershey's cocoa
1 9-inch pie shell, baked
¼ cup chopped peanuts

In a large bowl combine the Neufchâtel cheese, sugar, cocoa, and peanut butter.

In the bowl of an electric mixer whip the cream until soft peaks form. Fold the whipped cream into the peanut butter mixture. Pour the filling into the pie crust. Sprinkle chopped nuts over the surface. Place the pie in the freezer overnight. Allow the pie to soften slightly (about 20 minutes) before serving.

Serves 8

This Recipe

is LOW in HEME iron and contains the following substances that inhibit absorption of nonheme iron:

✓ calcium

✓ dairy phosphate

eggs

✓ phytate phosphorus

POLYPHENOLS

✓ tannic acid

✓ chlorogenic acid

phenolic acid

oxalates

Per Serving

IRON	heme iron	nonheme iron
	0.0 mg	0.8 mg

Pie Crust

2   cups flour
1   teaspoon salt
½   pound Crisco shortening
4   to 5 tablespoons cold skim milk

THIS RECIPE

is LOW in HEME iron and contains the following substances that inhibit absorption of nonheme iron:

✓ calcium

✓ dairy phosphate

eggs

✓ phytate phosphorus

POLYPHENOLS

tannic acid

chlorogenic acid

phenolic acid

oxalates

PER SERVING

IRON	heme iron	nonheme iron
	0.0 mg	1.17 mg

Place the flour and salt in a food processor. Pinch the shortening into pieces and drop into the flour. Pulse until blended. Gently add the cold milk a bit at a time, and pulse. Do not overprocess; the dough should stick together but should not be gooey. Remove and form into a smooth ball.

Tip: Wrap in waxed paper and refrigerate for 1 hour. The dough will be easier to handle.

Flour a pastry cloth. Separate the dough ball into 2 pieces, roll out, and line the baking dish with one crust. Use the second for the cover or refrigerate for another use.

Makes two 9-inch pie crusts

Plum Cake

2   cups whole-wheat flour
1   cup cocoa powder
1   teaspoon baking powder
2   teaspoons baking soda
¼   teaspoon salt
1⅔   cups sugar
10   ounces puréed plums
2   teaspoons vanilla extract
2   eggs
1   cup buttermilk
1   cup hot strong coffee
1   tablespoon instant coffee

GLAZE:
2   cups confectioners' sugar
¼   cup butter, melted
⅓   cup strong coffee

In a medium bowl sift the flour, cocoa, baking powder, baking soda, and salt together.

In a large bowl blend the sugar, puréed plums, vanilla, and eggs. Alternately add the flour mixture and the buttermilk and coffee. Stir the batter until blended.

Spray a rectangular baking dish generously with vegetable spray. Pour the batter into the prepared dish. Bake at 350° for 30 to 35 minutes until the center is done.

While still hot, poke holes in the cake. In a medium bowl combine the glaze ingredients and blend well. Pour the mixture over the surface of the cake and let cool.

Serves 8

THIS RECIPE

is LOW in HEME iron and contains the following substances that inhibit absorption of nonheme iron:

✓ calcium

✓ dairy phosphate

✓ eggs

✓ phytate phosphorus

POLYPHENOLS

✓ tannic acid

✓ chlorogenic acid

✓ phenolic acid

oxalates

PER SERVING

IRON	heme iron	nonheme iron
	0.0 mg	1.36 mg

The Hemochromatosis Cookbook

Raspberry Squares

3   cups oat blend flour
2   teaspoon baking powder
1   teaspoon salt
1   tablespoon instant tea
3   teaspoons sugar
1   cup (2 sticks) butter
½   cup olive oil
1   egg
⅔   cup raspberry jam
1   cup ground English walnuts

In a large bowl combine the flour, baking powder, salt, tea, and sugar. Cut in the butter with a fork or pastry cutter. Add the lightly beaten egg and the oil. The dough will be very stiff. Roll the dough into a rectangle ¼ inch thick.

Spray a cookie sheet with vegetable spray. Place the dough on cookie sheet and press the edges out so the dough covers the cookie sheet. Spread raspberry jam over the surface of the dough and sprinkle with ground nuts. Before baking, score the dough into 24 cookies using a pizza cutter. Bake at 350° for 12 to 15 minutes until the cookie is done.

Let stand 15 minutes before snapping the cookies apart.

Makes 24

THIS RECIPE

is LOW in HEME iron and contains the following substances that inhibit absorption of nonheme iron:

calcium
✓ dairy phosphate
✓ eggs
✓ phytate phosphorus
POLYPHENOLS
✓ tannic acid
✓ chlorogenic acid
✓ phenolic acid
oxalates

PER SERVING

IRON	heme iron	nonheme iron
	0.0 mg	0.8 mg

Spiced Apple Dessert Casserole

1/4	cup olive oil
3	cups whole-wheat bread crumbs
4	cups diced apples
1/4	cup apple juice
1/2	cup orange juice
1/4	cup sugar
1/4	teaspoon salt
1/2	teaspoon ground cloves
1/4	cup dry white wine

In a medium bowl combine the olive oil and bread crumbs. Set aside.

In a separate bowl mix the apples, juices, sugar, salt, cloves, and wine. Alternate layers of bread crumbs and apple mixture in an oiled 1-quart glass dish. Cover and bake at 350°. Uncover and bake an additional 15 to 20 minutes.

Serves 8

This Recipe

is LOW in HEME iron and contains the following substances that inhibit absorption of nonheme iron:

✓ calcium

✓ dairy phosphate

eggs

✓ phytate phosphorus

POLYPHENOLS

✓ tannic acid

✓ chlorogenic acid

✓ phenolic acid

oxalates

Per Serving

IRON	heme iron	nonheme iron
	0.0 mg	0.8 mg

Strawberry Jell-O Salad

1 cup hot green tea
1 6-ounce package strawberry Jell-O
1 10-ounce package frozen strawberries with liquid
1 6-ounce can crushed pineapple, drained
1 8-ounce package Neufchâtel cheese
½ cup cold apple juice
½ cup chopped English walnuts
¼ cup sour cream
1 tablespoon milk

Pour boiling hot tea over the gelatin and stir until the gelatin is dissolved. Add the frozen strawberries and pineapple.

Place the cream cheese in a food processor. Add the apple juice and pulse until runny. Add to the gelatin and fruit mixture. Fold in the nuts. Chill until set.

In a small bowl combine the sour cream and milk. Pour over the top of the set gelatin.

Serves 8

THIS RECIPE

is LOW in HEME iron and contains the following substances that inhibit absorption of nonheme iron:

✓ calcium

✓ dairy phosphate

eggs

✓ phytate phosphorus

POLYPHENOLS

✓ tannic acid

✓ chlorogenic acid

phenolic acid

oxalates

PER SERVING

IRON	heme iron	nonheme iron
	0.0 mg	0.7 mg

Strawberries and Cream Cake

1½ cups fresh Driscoll brand strawberries
1 3.4-ounce box Jell-O brand
   instant vanilla pudding
1½ cups cold milk
½ cup cold green tea
1 18¼-ounce box Duncan Hines
   brand yellow cake mix
1 pint heavy cream or nondairy
   topping

THIS RECIPE

*is LOW in HEME iron and contains
the following substances that
inhibit absorption of nonheme iron:*

✓ calcium

✓ dairy phosphate

✓ eggs

✓ phytate phosphorus

POLYPHENOLS

tannic acid

chlorogenic acid

phenolic acid

oxalates

PER SERVING

IRON	heme iron	nonheme iron
	0.0 mg	0.9 mg

Wash the strawberries and pat dry. Slice and stir into the pudding; reserve a few strawberries for garnish.

In a medium bowl combine the instant pudding, milk, and tea and mix as directed on the package. Chill until set.

Bake the yellow cake according to the instructions for 2 layers. Cool and split the layers. Spread a generous portion of pudding between the split layers but not on top.

In the bowl of an electric mixer whip the cream until stiff peaks form. Spread the cake with whipped topping. Refrigerate until served.

Serves 8

Sugar Cream Pie

½   cup butter
1   cup sugar
2   cups light cream
¼   cup cornstarch
¼   cup milk
1   9-inch pie shell, baked
¼   teaspoon nutmeg

THIS RECIPE

*is LOW in HEME iron and contains
the following substances that
inhibit absorption of nonheme iron:*

✓ calcium

✓ dairy phosphate

eggs

✓ phytate phosphorus

POLYPHENOLS

tannic acid

chlorogenic acid

phenolic acid

oxalates

PER SERVING

IRON	heme iron	nonheme iron
	0.0 mg	trace

Preheat oven to 400°.

In the top of a double boiler heat the butter, sugar, and cream until hot but not boiling.

In a container with a lid mix the cornstarch with the milk and shake vigorously. Pour into the butter mixture, stir, and continue cooking for 5 minutes. Pour the filling into the baked shell. Sprinkle nutmeg over the top. Bake at 400° for 5 to 6 minutes.

Refrigerate and serve chilled.

Serves 8

Glossary of Cooking Terms

Bake: To cook in a covered or uncovered container in an oven.

Barbecue: To cook on a rack or grill over hot charcoal or gas flame.

Baste: To cover cooking food, usually meat, with liquid such as broth for the purpose of adding flavor or moisture.

Beat: To make a mixture of ingredients, such as cake batter, smooth by adding air using a wooden spoon, wire whisk, or electric mixer.

Blanch: To preheat or precook in boiling water or steam, usually for the purpose of canning or preserving a food item for long-term storage such as freezing or canning.

Blend: To combine two or more separate ingredients, such as oil and vinegar until they become one.

Boil: To cook in water or broth until bubbles rise rapidly to the surface. To bring to a rolling boil is to cook on high temperature until bubbles rise rapidly and continually.

Braise: To cook slowly in a small amount of liquid or in steam in a covered pan. Also referred to as fricassee.

Bread: To coat meat or vegetables such as eggplant with bread or cracker crumbs, usually after dredging in flour and egg or soaking in buttermilk then coating with bread crumbs.

Broil: To cook at a high temperature where heat source is from above, such as in an oven.

Chop: To cut into smaller pieces with a sharp knife or food processor.

Combine: To mix two or more ingredients.

Cream: To mix one or more ingredients such as sugar and butter together until soft and creamy.

Cut in: To distribute fat such as shortening or butter, usually into flour, using a fork or specialty tool called a pastry blender. This can also be accomplished with a food processor and some mixers.

Dice: To cut into small cubes.

Dissolve: To combine a dry substance and a liquid, resulting in a solution.

Dredge: To coat or sprinkle with flour or other fine substance such as sugar.

Fold: To combine gently, usually using a rubber spatula or wire whisk, with two motions. One motion cuts vertically through the mixture and the other turns the mixture over by sliding the implement across the bottom of the mixing bowl.

Fry: To cook in fat.

Grate: To reduce to small particles or short string-like pieces by scraping a food item on a hand-held grate, or in a food processor. Commonly used for cheeses or spices and to make hash brown potatoes.

Knead: To manipulate with a pressing, turning, folding, and stretching motion, usually by hand or with a special mixer attachment. This process is used mostly in breadmaking.

Marinate: To allow food, usually meat, to stand in mixture of ingredients such as wine, herbs, honey, soy, etc., for a period of time, usually overnight so that added flavor can permeate food or to tenderize meat.

Mince: To cut or chop into small, fine pieces.

Mix: To combine two or more ingredients.

Parboil: To boil uncooked food until partially cooked, usually for the purpose of storage such as freezing.

Parch: To brown foods such as grains by means of dry heat.

Pasteurize: To preserve food, such as fruit juices, milk, and cheese, by heating to a temperature (140° to 180°F) that will destroy certain microorganisms and arrest fermentation.

Peel: To remove skins or the outer covering of fruits and vegetables.

Poach: To cook in hot water.

Puree: To force cooked food through a fine sieve, food mill, or to mix in a food processor, blender, or mixer until mixture is smooth and thick.

Reconstitute: To restore concentrated foods to their normal state, usually by adding water.

Reduce: To continue cooking a liquid until its volume is decreased, thickened or concentrated.

Rice: To force food through ricer, sieve, or food mill.

Roast: To cook by dry heat, usually in an oven in a roasting pan with a lid or in a roasting bag.

Sanitize: To clean with soap and water or bleach.

Sauté: To fry with a small amount of oil.

Sear: To brown meat quickly with intense heat.

Simmer: To cook in a liquid just below the boiling point.

Steam: To cook in a basket over hot, usually boiling water or in a pressure cooker.

Steep: To allow a substance, such as tea, to stand in liquid below the boiling point for the purpose of extracting flavor.

Sterilize: To destroy microorganisms usually with steam, dry heat, or by boiling in a liquid.

Stew: To cook slowly in a small amount of liquid.

Stir: To mix ingredients by hand, usually with a wooden spoon to avoid burning or to keep ingredients blended.

Tear: To pull apart by hand.

Whip: To rapidly beat air into foods such as eggs or heavy cream, to cause expansion.

Whisk: To combine ingredients, especially for sauces, with a wire whisk.

Cooking Tips

Health and Safety

Hot food should have a center temperature of 155 degrees, cold food a center temperature of 45 degrees.

White foods, such as pasta and rice, that are not properly cooled or fully reheated can provide the perfect environment for bacterial growth. All raw fruits and vegetables should be washed well before the skin is pierced. Melons, some berries, unpasteurized juices, and raw meat can contain E. coli bacteria. Handling these foods then touching other foods without thoroughly washing one's hands can lead to cross contamination of this potentially deadly bacteria.

Use of antibacterial soaps is not necessary; any hand soap or mild bleach will clean a countertop sufficiently to sanitize it for use. Allow the countertop to dry completely before using.

Substitutions and the Benefits of Using Brand Name Products

My mother always stressed the importance of using established brand-name products. She felt that these products offered consistency in cooking and especially in baking. Over the years I have come to agree with her; I have tried substitutions only to be disappointed. Some of my favorite brand names include:

Berio (olive oil), Breakstone (sour cream, cottage cheese, ricotta), Breyers (frozen yogurt, ice cream, and ice milk), Dannon (yogurt), Folger's Coffee (instant and classic brew), Heinz (ketchup and canned tomato products), Hellman's (mayonnaise), Jell-O (gelatins and puddings), JIF (peanut butter), Keebler (crackers), Kellogg's Complete Oat Bran, Kraft (cheeses and cheese products and some prepared salad dressings), Kikkoman (soy or teriyaki sauce), Lipton (tea), Nestle's and Hershey's (chocolate), Post Shredded Wheat Mini with Wheat Bran, Uncle Ben's (rice), Quaker Oats, and Ovaltine.

More recently, I have found that some store brands are actually the same product as the highly marketed name brand. It is worth experimenting with various brands, especially when a brand provides more beneficial levels of fats, carbs, proteins, or fillers.

Low-Fat Tips and Good Substitutions

Sour cream and mayonnaise are two fats that are prevalent in the American diet. In *The Hemochromatosis Cookbook*, sour cream especially is used in several recipes because of its iron-inhibiting characteristics. However, caution is advised with respect to the frequency one consumes these fats. Use of fat-free products offers some reduction in fat, but often fat-free versions are high in sugar and sodium. One solution is to limit the number of times recipes with sour cream or mayonnaise are selected. Another approach is to use reduced-fat products that you make yourself. Refer to reduced-fat recipes such as mayonnaise and sour cream (see intro to Sauces chapter), "faux" bacon, and salad dressing (see the index for choices).

Thickening agent: 1 tablespoon cornstarch = 2 tablespoons flour.

Vinegar: Substitute lemon juice.

Buttermilk: 1 cup sweet milk plus 1 tablespoon vinegar.

Table salt: No Salt by RCN Products or Morton's Lite Salt. Both products can leave a slightly bitter aftertaste when used in recipes that stand for a while. Lite Salt, was less bitter. Both taste fine in cooked or baked foods. Use these products as needed rather than using them in products prepared ahead.

Sugar substitute: Stevia (*Stevia rebaudiana*) is non-caloric herb that is several times more sweet than white table sugar; only a couple of drops in a beverage is required to reach the same sweet level as other sweeteners. It is readily available in health food stores and may be available in the specialty foods section of the grocery store. Stevia has a slightly bitter aftertaste and the side effects are not fully known. The FDA banned its use as an artificial sweetener in the early 90s, but later approved its use as a supplement. Most reports about Stevia by scientific investigators conclude that it is safe consumption. One study performed on rats fed steviocide (powder form of Stevia) demonstrated that steviocide generated lesions in peripheral blood, liver, brain, and spleen cells in different levels, the largest effect being in the liver. Hemochromatosis diabetes patients report that they do very well with Stevia. There are no known scientific studies about changes to composition of Stevia when used in cooking.

Milk: Vitamite® nondairy beverage. This is a personal favorite of mine. I use it in my coffee and on cereal; it tastes just like milk to me. Anyone who is allergic to dairy might want to try this product. Vitamite cooks well, except that it will not thicken instant puddings—you will need to add 1 teaspoon of cornstarch dissolved in a bit of water to your instant pudding recipes. If you cannot find Vitamite in stores, contact the manufacturers through the website www.diehlinc.com/home.html.

Equivalents

3 teaspoons = 1 tablespoon

4 tablespoons = ¼ cup

5 tablespoons + 1 teaspoon = ⅓ cup

2 cups = 1 pint

2 pints = 1 quart

4 quarts = 1 gallon

1 ounce = 2 tablespoons

8 ounces = 1 cup

16 ounces = 1 pound

Diet Success Stories from People Living with Hemochromatosis

Jane Depew's iron story began when she was diagnosed with hemochromatosis at the age of sixty-four by a family doctor. He had recently read an article about hemochromatosis and ordered tests for Jane. Even though genetic testing revealed that she was a C282Y/C282Y homozygote, except for minor knee discomfort, Jane did not have symptoms of HHC. Nor were her iron levels all that high. Still, she began phlebotomies at the recommendation of her doctor. On a routine follow-up Jane was told that she was prediabetic and at risk for developing full-blown diabetes if she did not get her blood sugar under control. Not wanting to be on medication, Jane asked how she could control her blood sugar. "Lose 50 pounds!" was her doctor's response as he handed her a large stack of literature about diabetes and blood sugar control.

Jane was already conditioned to watch her iron levels, which had become too low. She was iron avid. Now she had to incorporate a diet plan to get her iron levels back up to normal *and* keep the blood sugar under control. Jane's first step was to immediately cut out all sugar. She also began reading everything she could find on diabetes and iron. She was looking for a simple plan, one that she could stick to. She knew if the plan was too complicated she would give up.

With the help of Iron Disorders Institute, it took Jane two years to bring her iron levels back into balance. To manage her diabetes, she found an approach that worked for her, one that included exercise, nutritional label reading, planning meals ahead, and noting the protein, carb, fat, and iron content of everything she consumed. She aimed for a 1:1 ratio of carbs to protein, eating smaller portions more frequently throughout the day, something she had learned was important from her reading. Her key resources remain the American Diabetes Association Food Exchange booklet, *The Insulin Resistance Diet*, and the Iron Disorders Institute patient support services.

In just under a year her weight is under control; she has lost seventy-five pounds. She warns against too many combination foods, such as lasagna, and stresses the importance of taking charge of own's own health by reading and utilizing the many resources available.

Chip Sullivan's iron story began in 2004. One of his sisters had been very ill and eventually lost her battle, dying at the age of forty-four from diabetes and liver failure due to hemochromatosis. At the time, it did not seem possible to Chip that he might also be at risk for hemochromatosis since he was an active golfer and by all appearances healthy. But within two years of his sister's death, Chip displayed symptoms of chronic fatigue. Not long after, Chip got his diagnosis: diabetes and hemochromatosis, the same diagnosis that had led to his sister's premature death.

Most of the dietary changes Chip made were for the diabetes. Regular phlebotomies helped to lower his iron levels, but because sugar increases absorption of iron, his reduction of sugar consumption was beneficial to controlling not only his blood sugar but also the rate he absorbed iron. Chip drinks more water, which helps him stay hydrated for the phlebotomies. He chooses sugar-free or diet drinks rather than regular soft drinks. Chip has also eliminated starchy foods such as potatoes, chips, and French-fries from his diet. These foods convert to sugar quickly. Fries and chips usually are prepared in fats that should be avoided by hemochromatosis patients. Fats in combination with unbound iron can trigger free radical activity, which causes cell destruction. So ironically, the diet Chip needs to control his diabetes is a good diet for his hemochromatosis also. Chip's victory over these two potentially deadly diseases was highlighted when he won the 2007 Professional Golfer's Association (PGA) National Championship.

Harry Kieffer's iron story began at the age of forty-nine. His serum ferritin was 2960 and his transferrin-iron saturation percentage (TS%) was 98 percent! Harry was especially watchful of his iron intake during phlebotomies. He recalls, "It seemed logical that if I needed to remove iron then I should take in less of it so as not to prolong my treatments. My wife had read a lot about iron, and we adjusted our diets accordingly, eliminating spinach and other high-iron foods. After calling a scientist at NIH (National Institutes of Health), we once again started eating vegetables that contained iron. The scientist explained that vegetable and fruit sources of iron were not as readily available to the body as beef. The scientist also told my wife that I should eat a balanced diet. We reduced our red meat intake tremendously, which was good because that was the biggest source of iron to the body. We had already changed our breakfast cereal from our favorite, Special K, to a low-fortified one, and avoided orange juice with breakfast as well. Our stress-formula daily vitamin with extra iron was a very bad choice. For the previous seven years, we had thought we were being good to ourselves by taking this daily vitamin, but we had, in fact, compounded my problems. My wife then called Tetley Tea and spoke with a scientist who confirmed that the tannins in tea blocked iron absorption. She questioned if the decaffeinating process also might remove the valuable tannins. She was told it did not! So we increased tea consumption. I also traveled a lot and enjoyed raw oysters. Looking back at my high iron levels, I guess I am lucky to be alive with the bacteria raw oysters sometimes contain—what I was eating could have killed me. When I was diagnosed fifteen years ago, we could find very little information about this iron-loading disorder, especially about diet. We didn't have a computer and knew little of the Internet. A book like this one would have made life easier."

Art Callahan set off metal detectors in airports for years before he was diagnosed with an inherited iron-loading condition called G6PD deficiency. Glucose 6 phosphate dehydrogenase (G6PD) is an enzyme deficiency more prevalent in males than females. It is one of several anemias where iron overload can be a consequence. Persons with G6PD are prone to hemolysis (red blood cell destruction), which leads to iron overload. Once diagnosed, Art found that certain antibiotics, sinus medication, and alcohol made his condition flare up. He was also told that eating fava beans could trigger an episode of hemolysis. Art's serum ferritin at time of diagnosis was over 1,500 with an accompanying saturation percentage of 70 percent. He began treatment but after removal of 20 pints of blood, his ferritin level only dropped to 1,390 and his saturation percentage remained well above 50 percent. Art decided that diet changes must be made. He decided to stick to a low-iron diet and to make every effort to limit the amount of iron absorbed. Art says, "I consider my G6PD hemolytic anemia much different and more complex than hemochromatosis. Iron disorder treatments are similar but phlebotomy rates and frequency and iron absorption rates differ with each individual. Some people may not think diet is important. I had a physician tell me that diet wouldn't matter in my case, but I have learned that diet is a big deal. I believe a low-iron diet has to be adhered to in my case. I think a book like *The Hemochromatosis Cookbook* would be helpful for *anyone* at risk for iron overload."

David Garrison's iron story began when he was just sixteen. He had symptoms of joint pain, profound fatigue, enlarged spleen, and very high iron levels. He had lost forty pounds within two months; his skin was an ashen gray green. His blood sugar was elevated and so was his iron. "Wildly high" was noted by the doctor next to the fasting serum iron lab test report. David does not have the genes for classic hemochromatosis; he is a carrier of the H63D mutation. "I have an iron-loading disorder, but doctors can't figure out why. I don't have the typical gene mutations for hemochromatosis. Also my iron-loading condition showed up when I was only sixteen, which is unusual for people with HHC. But I do load iron and have to have phlebotomies to keep my iron levels normal. I also learned what I ate would have an impact on how often I had to donate blood. In the beginning I thought my mom was just being a typical mom when she kept reminding me to cut back on burgers and watch the high vitamin C drinks. After several years of learning how my body responds to iron and seeing for myself that I can control to some extent how much iron I absorb by watching what I eat, I am now more careful. When I ate mostly junk food and drank sodas or orange juice almost exclusively, I needed a phlebotomy more often. When I learned about iron bioavailability and how to block absorption I began cooking my own food. I changed the way I ate and found that I could go longer between phlebotomies. It is important to know that I don't drink alcohol or smoke, which can add to the problem. By the way, after my first few phlebotomies, my blood sugar level went back down to normal and has remained normal."

Jen Opperman found out that she was a compound heterozygote (two different mutations of the hemochromatosis gene HFE) after years of infertility, depression, and pain. Doctors had told her hereditary hemochromatosis was rare and didn't affect females. Jen proved otherwise. She eventually received treatment (phlebotomy) and was deironed. She was now anemic, but fearing her iron-loading condition would cause iron to build back up in her system she decided to reduce the amount of iron she consumed. Jen cut out all meat, wine, supplements, and vitamin C–rich foods and juices. To her surprise her ferritin levels began to drop as though she were having periodic phlebotomies. (It must be noted that persons with iron-loading conditions whose tissue iron levels are very high, warranting phlebotomy, cannot efficiently reduce iron levels. In Jen's case, she was mildly anemic and her iron stores depleted as a result of blood removal. Jen soon learned by experimentation that she did not need such extreme dietary changes.) Her maintenance needed balance in her diet. Jen started including more iron-rich foods in her diet and her iron levels began to rise. She eventually needed another phlebotomy but has learned the importance of caution and balance in diet. "People can go to extreme," says Jen. "I did, because my doctors just didn't understand diet and iron overload. I think this cookbook is an important book for anyone striving to keep iron levels in balance. Ironically, symptoms that resulted from my self-induced anemia were almost as bad as the symptoms of iron overload."

Contacts

For more information about hereditary hemochromatosis, iron overload, and other disorders of iron contact:

Iron Disorders Institute
P.O. Box 675
Taylors, SC 29687
Toll Free: 888-565-4766 (IRON)
www.irondisorders.org
www.hemochromatosis.org

An excellent resource: *The Iron Disorders Institute Guide to Hemochromatosis*—available in major bookstores.

For more information about nutrition, diet, and dietary supplements visit the following websites:

http://arborcom.com/frame/arb_food.htm
http://sun.kent.wednet.edu/KSD/KR/APPLIED/HEALTH/nutrition_values.html
http://www.cdc.gov (search with words *nutrition* and *hemochromatosis*)
http://dietary-supplements.info.nih.gov/
http://www.nal.usda.gov/fnic/foodcomp/
http://www.nih.gov (search with words *nutrition* and *hemochromatosis*)
http://www.nutritionfocus.com/
http://diabetes.niddk.nih.gov/dm/pubs/eating_ez/index.htm
    This site provides excellent illustrations and includes "What I Need to Know About Eating and Diabetes."
http://www.cdc.gov/diabetes/

Bibliography and Resources

Al-Waili, N. S. "Effects of Daily Consumption of Honey Solution on Hematological Indices and Blood Levels of Minerals and Enzymes in Normal Individuals." *Journal of Medicinal Food* 6 (2003): 135–40.

Ann-Sofie Sandberg, Mats Brune, Nils-Gunnar Carlsson, Leif Hallberg, Erika Skoglund, and Lena Rossander-Hulthén. "Inositol Phosphates with Different Numbers of Phosphate Groups Influence Iron Absorption in Humans." *American Journal of Clinical Nutrition*, 70 (1999): 240–46.

Barton, J. C., S. M. McDonnell, P. C. Adams, P. Brissot, L. W. Powell, C. Q. Edwards, J. D. Cook, and K. V. Kowdle. "Management of Hemochromatosis." *Annals Internal Medicine* 129 (1998): 932–39.

Beard, J., and B. Tobin. "Iron Status and Exercise." *American Journal of Clinical Nutrition* 72 (2001): S594–97.

Bendich. A. "Calcium Supplementation and Iron Status of Females." *Nutrition* 17 (2001): 46–51.

Bothwell, T. H., R. D. Baynes, B. J. MacFarlane, and A. P. MacPhail. "Nutritional Iron Requirements and Food Iron Absorption." *Journal of Internal Medicine* 226 (1989): 357–65.

Cook, J. D., and C. A. Finch. "Assessing Iron Status of a Population." *American Journal of Clinical Nutrition* 32 (1979): 2115–19.

Cook, J. D., and E. R. Monsen. "Comparison of the Effect of Animal Proteins on Nonheme Iron Absorption." *American Journal of Clinical Nutrition* 29 (1976): 859–67.

Cook, J. D., and M. B. Reddy. "Ascorbic Acid Has a Pronounced Enhancing Effect on the Absorption of Dietary Nonheme Iron when Assessed by Feeding Single Meals to Fasting Subjects." *American Journal of Clinical Nutrition* 73 (2001): 93–8.

Davidsson, L., T. Walczyk, N. Zavaleta, and R. F. Hurrell. "Improving Iron Absorption from a Peruvian School Breakfast Meal by Adding Ascorbic Acid or Na(2)EDTA." *American Journal of Clinical Nutrition* 73 (2001): 283–87.

Duane P., K. B. Raja, R. J. Simpson, and T. J. Peters. "Intestinal Iron Absorption in Chronic Alcoholism." *Alcohol Alcoholism* 27 (1992): 539–44.

Fleming, D. J., P. F. Jacques, K. L. Tucker, J. M. Massaro, R. B. D'Agostino Sr, P. W. Wilson, and R. J. Wood. "Iron Status of the Free-living, Elderly Framingham

Heart Study Cohort: An Iron-replete Population with a High Prevalence of Elevated Iron Stores." *American Journal of Clinical Nutrition* 73 (2001): 638–46.

Fleming, D. J., K. L. Tucker, P. F. Jacques, G. E. Dallal, P. W., Wilson, and R. J. Wood. "Dietary Factors Associated with the Risk of High Iron Stores in the Elderly Framingham Heart Study Cohort." *American Journal of Clinical Nutrition* 76 (2002): 1375–84.

Garcia-Casal, M. N., I. Leets, and M. Layrisse. "Beta-Carotene and Inhibitors of Iron Absorption Modify Iron Uptake by Caco-2 Cell." *Journal of Nutrition* 130 (2000): 5–9.

Griffin, I., S. Abrams. "Iron and Breastfeeding." *The Management of Breastfeeding* 48 (2001): 401–13.

Hallberg, L, and L. Hulthén. "Prediction of Dietary Iron Absorption: An Algorithm for Calculating Absorption and Bioavailability of Dietary Iron." *American Journal of Clinical Nutrition* 71 (2000): 1147–60.

Han, O., M. L. Failla, A. D. Hill, E. R. Morris, and J. C. Smith Jr. "Inositol Phosphates Inhibit Uptake and Transport of Iron and Zinc by a Human Intestinal Cell Line." *Journal of Nutrition* 124 (1994): 580–87.

Harnly, J. M., R. F. Doherty, G. R. Beecher, J. M. Holden, D. B. Haytowitz, S. Bhagwat, and S. Gebhardt. "Flavonoid Content of U.S. Fruits, Vegetables, and Nuts." *Journal of Agriculture and Food Chemistry* 54 (2006): 9966–77.

Heath, A. L., C. M. Skeaff, and R. S. Gibson. "The Relative Validity of a Computerized Food Frequency Questionnaire for Estimating Intake of Dietary Iron and Its Absorption Modifiers." *European Journal of Clinical* Nutrition 54 (2000): 592–99.

Hunt, J. R., Z. K. Roughead. "Nonheme Iron Absorption, Fecal Ferritin Excretion, and Blood Indexes of Iron Status in Women Consuming Controlled Lactoovovegetarian Diets for Eight Weeks." *American Journal of Clinical Nutrition* 69 (1999): 944–52.

Hurrell, R. F., M. Reddy, and J. D. Cook. "Inhibition of Non-haem Iron Absorption in Man by Polyphenolic-containing Beverages." *British Journal of Nutrition* 81 (1999): 289–95.

Hurrell, R. F., M. B. Reddy, J. Burri, and J. D. Cook. "An Evaluation of EDTA Compounds for Iron Fortification of Cereal-based Foods." *British Journal of Nutrition* 84 (2000): 903–10.

Kaltwasser, J. P., E. Werner, K. Schalk, C. Hansen, R. Gottschalk, and C. Seidl. "Clinical Trial on the Effect of Regular Tea Drinking on Iron Accumulation in Genetic Haemochromatosis." *Gut* 43 (1998): 699–704.

Kamao, M., N. Tsugawa, K. Nakagawa, Y. Kawamoto, K. Fukui, K. Takamatsu, G. Kuwata, M. Imai, and T. Okano. "Absorption of Calcium, Magnesium, Phosphorus, Iron and Zinc in Growing Male Rats Fed Diets Containing Either Phytate-free Soybean Protein or Soybean Protein Isolate or Casein." *Journal of Nutrition Science Vitaminol* (Tokyo) 46 (2000): 34–41.

Kishida, T., Y. Nakai, and Ebihara K. "Hydroxypropyl-Distarch Phosphate from Tapioca Starch Reduces Zinc and Iron Absorption, but Not Calcium and Magnesium Absorption in Rats." *Journal of Nutrition* 131 (2001): 294–300.

Layrisse, M., C. Martinez-Torres, M. Renzi, F. Velez, and M. Gonzalez. "Sugar as a Vehicle for Iron Fortification." *American Journal of Clinical Nutrition* 29 (1976): 8–18.

Layrisse, M., M. Garcia-Casal, L. Solano, M. Baron, F. Arguello, D. Llovera, J. Ramierz, I. Leets, and E. Tropper. "Iron Bioavailability in Humans from Breakfasts Enriched with Iron Bis-Glycine Chelate, Phytates and Polyphenols." *Human Nutrition and Metabolism* 9 (2000): 2195–99.

Levrat-Verny, M. A., C. Coudray, J. Bellanger, H. W. Lopez, C. Demigne, Y. Rayssiguier, and C. Remesy. "Wholewheat Flour Ensures Higher Mineral Absorption and Bioavailability than White Wheat Flour in Rats." *British Journal of Nutrition* 82 (1999): 17–21.

Mallory, M. A., C. Sthapanachai, and K. V. Kowdley. "Iron Overload Related to Excessive Vitamin C Intake."*Annals Internal Medicine* 139(6) (2003): 532–33.

Morck, T. A., S. R. Lynch, and J. D. Cook. "Inhibition of Food Iron Absorption by Coffee." *The American Journal of Clinical Nutrition* 37 (1983): 416–20.

Passwater, R. A. *Beta-Carotene: The Backstage Nutrient Now Universally Recognized for Cancer Prevention*. New Canaan, Connecticut: Keats Publishing Inc., 1984.

Pruchnicki, M. C., J. D. Coyle, S. Hoshaw-Woodard, and W. H. Bay. "Effect of Phosphate Binders on Supplemental Iron Absorption in Healthy Subjects." *Journal of Clinical Pharmacology* 42(10) (2002): 1171–76.

Roughead, Z. K., C. A. Zito, and J. R. Hunt. "Initial Uptake and Absorption of Nonheme Iron and Absorption of Heme Iron in Humans are Unaffected by the Addition of Calcium as Cheese to a Meal with High Iron Bioavailability." *American Journal Clinical Nutrition* 76(2) (2002): 419–25.

Roughead, Z. K., and J. R. Hunt. "Adaptation in Iron Absorption: Iron Supplementation Reduces Nonheme-Iron but Not Heme-Iron Absorption from Food." *American Journal of Clinical Nutrition* 72 (2000): 982–89.

Sandstead, H. H. "Causes of Iron and Zinc Deficiencies and their Effects on Brain." *Journal of Nutrition* 130 (2000): 347S-349S.Siegenberg, D., R. D. Baynes, T. H. Bothwell, B. J. MacFarlane, R. D. Lamparelli, N. G. Car, P. MacPhail, U. Schmidt, A. Tal, and F. Mayet. "Ascorbic Acid Prevents the Dose-Dependent Inhibitory Effects of Polyphenols and Phytates on Nonheme-iron Absorption." *American Journal of Clinical Nutrition* 53 (1991): 537–41.

Wu, C, H., Y. C. Yang, W. J. Yan, F. H. Lu, J. S. Wu, and C. J. Chang. "Epidemiological Evidence on Increased Bone Mineral Density in Habitual Tea Drinkers." *Archives Internal Medicine* 162 (2002): 1001–6.

Zijp, I. M., O. Korver, and L. B. Tijburg. "Effect of Tea and Other Dietary Factors on Iron Absorption." *Critical Review Food Science & Nutrition* 40 (2000): 371–98.

Subject Index

Recipe Index